LEFT VENTRICULAR HYPERTROPHY (LVH)

PREVALENCE, RISK FACTORS AND TREATMENT

CARDIOLOGY RESEARCH AND CLINICAL DEVELOPMENTS

CARDIOLOGY RESEARCH AND CLINICAL DEVELOPMENTS

LEFT VENTRICULAR HYPERTROPHY (LVH)

PREVALENCE, RISK FACTORS AND TREATMENT

RICHARD T. MATTHEWS

EDITOR

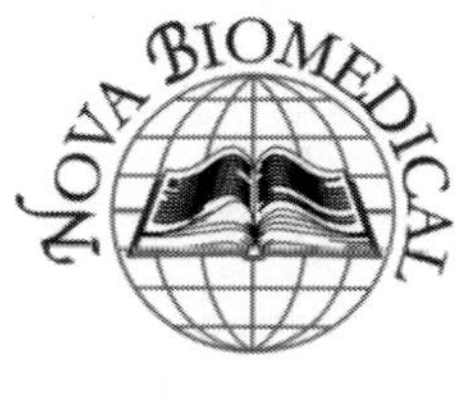

NOVA BIOMEDICAL

New York

Library of Congress Cataloging-in-Publication Data

ISBN: 978-1-63463-022-1
Library of Congress Control Number: 2014950572

Published by Nova Science Publishers, Inc. † New York

Contents

Preface

This book discusses the prevalence, risk factors and treatment options available for LVH.

Chapter 1 - Left Ventricular Hypertrophy (LVH) is defined as an increase in the left ventricular mass. Hypertrophy is a physiologic response to the increased wall stress from hemodynamic overload. The physiological changes become pathological with deleterious effects when the stress is prolonged. Genetic and infiltrative disorders have also been associated with hypertrophy, but will not be discussed in this chapter. The risk factors associated with increase in wall stress can be classified as: pressure vs. volume overload and concentric vs. eccentric hypertrophy (based on the type of hypertrophy in response to the stressor). Prevalence depends on the modality and criteria used for diagnosis and studies have shown varying results. LVH has also been reported to be more frequent in certain non-cardiac disease conditions like chronic kidney disease, anemia and obesity.

The pathophysiology behind the development of LVH is complex and involves gene re-programming induced by the mechanical stimuli via electro-mechanical transducers in the cell surface accompanied with G-protein coupled neuro-hormones. Other signaling molecules and changes in the connective tissue matrix have also been proposed in the pathogenesis.

Though LVH is not a disease process per se, it can have varied clinical implications like diastolic dysfunction, systolic dysfunction, myocardial ischemia, arrhythmia and sudden cardiac death. Diastolic dysfunction is the most common clinical implication and contributes to heart failure with preserved ejection fraction. Identification and proper treatment institution are of paramount importance as they have >4 fold risk of death compared to the general population. Non cardiac factors have also been reported to increase the risk of diastolic dysfunction in patients with LVH. Atrial fibrillation is the most common supraventricular arrhythmia associated with LVH.

Value of clinical examination in the diagnosis of LVH in patients without any complications is limited. Though echocardiogram is one of the gold standard investigation, the inexpensive and easily available electrocardiogram (EKG) is the most commonly used modality. The most common abnormalities noticed in EKG are increased QRS voltage and duration, leftward axis, left atrial abnormality and repolarization abnormalities. Multiple criteria have been proposed for the diagnosis. The sensitivity and specificity depends on the criterion used. Studies have shown that use of multiple criteria has improved the diagnostic accuracy. Non-cardiac confounders have also been reported to affect the sensitivity and specificity of the criteria. Separate criteria for computer based interpretations have been proposed based on regression models. Apart from the diagnosis, EKG is also useful in prognostication. Regression of EKG changes of LVH with treatment of underlying factors, has been shown to correlate with reduction in risk for adverse cardiovascular outcomes. American Society of echocardiography has proposed guidelines for the diagnosis of LVH by echocardiogram.

Treatment of LVH is primarily targeted at the causative factors. Complete normalization of LVH has been shown in patients, who had the corrective measures for the mechanical problem causing the increased wall stress. However, this near normal reversal is not seen with treatment of hypertension. The degree of reversal has been shown to correlate with adequacy of control and also the agent used for therapy. Complications secondary to LVH should be managed based on the problems and attempts should be made to preserve sinus rhythm and avoid tachycardia for better outcomes. Regression of LVH with adequate treatment has been shown to decrease the cardiovascular risk significantly. In case of CKD, maintenance of hemoglobin between 10 to 12 grams/dl has shown reduction in left ventricular mass index and improved outcomes.

Chapter 2 - Aortic valve stenosis is the most common valvular heart disease in the Western world. It currently affects more than 7% of the population over the age of 60, with severe stenosis affecting in excess of 3% of people over the age of 75. In parallel with an aging population, the prevalence of aortic stenosis and need for surgery are expected to double over the next 20 years increasing further the burden on healthcare resources.

Left untreated aortic stenosis leads to an abnormally high pressure load on the left ventricle, a pathological process that induces myocyte hypertrophy and fibrosis. Initially, the adaptive process of increased wall thickness maintains normal wall stress, contraction and cardiac output. However, ultimately this becomes maladaptive leading to ventricular stiffness, an increase in myocyte hypertrophy and myocardial fibrosis eventually causing diastolic and systolic dysfunction and increased morbidity and mortality.

At present there is no effective medical therapy capable of altering this course and aortic valve intervention, usually in the form of surgical aortic valve replacement, is recommended by international guidelines in patients with severe stenosis and evidence of LV decompensation (either on the basis of symptoms or a reduced ejection fraction). Following aortic valve intervention patients demonstrate a variable degree of regression of the ventricular hypertrophy with favorable prognosis demonstrated in the cohort of patients with the highest level of regression.

In this chapter the authors will discuss the prevalence and mechanism of left ventricular hypertrophy, fibrosis and decompensation in patients with aortic stenosis. Through case examples the authors will illustrate common cases of patients with hypertrophy relating to AS and analyze the most recent guidelines from the American Heart Association/American College of Cardiology (2014) and European Society of Cardiology (2012) on managing patients with aortic stenosis.

Chapter 3 - Cardiovascular diseases such as coronary artery disease, congestive heart failure, arrhtyhmias and sudden cardiac death represent main causes of morbidity and mortality in patients with chronic kidney disease (CKD). Pathogenesis includes close linkage between heart and kidneys and involves traditional and non-traditional risk factors. According to well – established classification of cardio – renal syndrome, cardiovascular involvement in chronic kidney disease is known as "Type 4 Cardio – Renal Syndrome" (chronic reno – cardiac).

Uremic cardiopathy is mainly characterized by both left ventricular systolic and diastolic impairment, often associated to right heart dysfunction due to presence of vascular access for hemodialysis.

Typical clinical picture is represented by left ventricular hypertrophy (LVH), which pathogenesis is multifactorial and closely linked to elevated blood pressure, vascular stiffness and atherosclerosis.

Diagnosis is mainly provided by ultrasound (2D and 3D echocardiography) and cardiac magnetic resonance imaging (CMRI), although echocardiography is most widely employed because it's non – invasive and cheaper than CMRI.

Following chapter makes an overview about epidemiology, pathophysiology, diagnosis and treatment key features of left ventricular hypertrophy CKD patients

Chapter 4 - Left ventricular hypertrophy (LVH) is prevalent and carries poor prognosis. Although the relative risk of cardiovascular mortality increases with incremental left ventricular mass, many underlying causes are reversible if timely treatment is instigated.

The authors discuss the clinical definition and diagnostic criteria of LVH, its prevalence, risk factors and treatment. A pragmatic systematic approach is adopted for targeted assessment and investigations of the common (hypertension, valvular heart disease, obesity, athletic heart) and rare (inherited, infiltrative and metabolic cardiomyopathies) underlying causes of LVH.

Chapter 5 - The aim of this study is to assess whether carotid lesion might reflect preclinical target organ damage (TOD) and its relationship with cardiac remodeling in hypertension in aging. Patients (n=93) underwent electro- and echocardiographic evaluation, 24-hr Holter recording, BP monitoring, pulse wave velocity (PWV) determinations and routine analyses. Carotid damage was associated with an increase in diurnal and nocturnal systolic BP variability (BPVar) even after controlling for age, sex and body mass index. Eccentric remodeling was related to diastolic BPVar ($p<0.05$), diurnal systolic BPVar ($p<0.02$) and plaque atheroma development ($p<0.001$). Concentric remodeling was related to PWV variation ($p<0.03$). Patients with left ventricle hypertrophy showed higher prevalence of carotid atheroma (62% vs 33% normal geometry, $p<0.01$). The relationship between carotid damage and increased BPVar suggests a role for the former as a sign of preclinical TOD. Cardiac geometry might prove a reliable indicator of cardiovascular risk in hypertension in aging.

Chapter 6 - *Background:* Currently, left ventricular (LV) hypertrophy and dysfunction are considered to be the strongest predictors of cardiovascular mortality in chronic kidney disease (CKD) patients. The authors investigated the factors associated with elevated LV mass index (LVMI) using echocardiography and assessed the therapeutic implications of strategies used to treat CKD (stages 1–5D) patients.

Methods: The authors prospectively determined correlations among biochemical values, physical specimens, and LVMI using echocardiography in 30 nondiabetic hemodialysis (HD) and 32 peritoneal dialysis (PD) (stage 5D) patients. These parameters were measured at 0 (baseline), 12, and 24 months after initiation of dialysis. Physical, biochemical, and LVMI data evaluated using echocardiography were also retrospectively analyzed in 930 CKD (stages 1–5) patients.

Results: In HD patients, LVMI values at 12 and 24 months were not significantly decreased compared with those at baseline. Systolic blood pressure (SBP), residual glomerular filtration rate, and serum albumin levels at baseline were identified as independent risk factors for LVMI in multivariate regression analysis. In PD patients, LVMI values at 12 and 24 months were significantly decreased compared with those at baseline (p < 0.05). Plasma atrial natriuretic peptide (ANP) was significantly correlated with left atrium diameter (LAD) and LVMI. In CKD (stages 4–5) patients, SBP, serum albumin levels, and left atrium volume index measured using echocardiography were identified as independent risk factors for duration before initiation of dialysis on multivariate regression analysis. In CKD (stage 1–5) patients, LVMI increased with decreasing renal function. Levels of SBP and hemoglobin (Hb) were independent risk factors for LVMI in the multivariate regression analysis. In the patients who showed worsening LVMI, the rates of change in SBP, proteinuria, and Hb were identified as independent risk factors for LVMI changes.

Conclusions: It is difficult to improve LVH in HD patients. Plasma ANP and LAD measurements showed that left ventricular structure, contraction, and compliance were well preserved in PD patients undergoing aggressive treatment. It is important to treat hypertension and overhydration on the basis of plasma ANP and Hb levels before initiating dialysis. The author's findings may have some therapeutic implications for the strategies used to treat predialysis and dialysis patients.

Chapter 7 - Left ventricular hypertrophy (LVH) accompanies the altered energy metabolism of the heart, and the altered energetics is hypothesized to play an important role in the progression of heart failure. However, the mechanism underlying these changes, and whether these changes are beneficial or detrimental, are not known because simultaneous evaluation of multiple metabolites is difficult and substrates in perfusion buffer are limited in ex vivo perfused heart experiments. Metabolomics is an emerging field of study, which uses mass spectrometry and/or nuclear magnetic resonance. This enables the monitoring of hundreds of metabolites from tissues or body fluids, and facilitates the identification of various metabolites simultaneously, and helps evaluate global changes in metabolites levels during cellular and physiological responses to external stimuli. The metabolomic analysis of an animal model with hypertensive LVH and decompensated heart failure indicates significant changes in cardiac energy metabolism. In human studies, metabolomics has been used to analyze blood or heart tissue samples from patients with cardiovascular diseases, such as ischemic heart disease, atrial fibrillation, ischemia reperfusion, heart failure, and metabolic syndrome. These reports not only provide significant information on the underlying mechanism of these diseases but also suggest potential biomarkers for the diagnosis of these conditions. Coupling metabolomics with other approaches, such as functional genomics and proteomics, can help determine the pathophysiology of cardiovascular diseases, discover biomarkers, and identify targets for therapeutic intervention.

ISBN: 978-1-63463-022-1
© 2015 Nova Science Publishers, Inc.

Chapter 1

Left Ventricular Hypertrophy: A Comprehensive Clinical Review

---

*Ramprakash Devadoss[1], M.D., Priyamvada Singh[1], M.D. and Lovely Chhabra[*2], M.D.*
[1]Dept. of Medicine, Saint Vincent Hospital, Worcester, Massachusetts, US
[2]Dept. of Cardiology, Hartford Hospital,
University of Connecticut School of Medicine, Hartford, Connecticut, US

Abstract

Left Ventricular Hypertrophy (LVH) is defined as an increase in the left ventricular mass. Hypertrophy is a physiologic response to the increased wall stress from hemodynamic overload. The physiological changes become pathological with deleterious effects when the stress is prolonged. Genetic and infiltrative disorders have also been associated with hypertrophy, but will not be discussed in this chapter. The risk factors associated with increase in wall stress can be classified as: pressure vs. volume overload and concentric vs. eccentric hypertrophy (based on the type of hypertrophy in response to the stressor). Prevalence depends on the modality and criteria used for diagnosis and studies have shown varying results. LVH has also been reported to be more frequent in certain non-cardiac disease conditions like chronic kidney disease, anemia and obesity.

The pathophysiology behind the development of LVH is complex and involves gene re-programming induced by the mechanical stimuli via electro-mechanical transducers in the cell surface accompanied with G-protein coupled neuro-hormones. Other signaling molecules and changes in the connective tissue matrix have also been proposed in the pathogenesis.

Though LVH is not a disease process per se, it can have varied clinical implications like diastolic dysfunction, systolic dysfunction, myocardial ischemia, arrhythmia and sudden cardiac death. Diastolic dysfunction is the most common clinical implication and contributes to heart failure with preserved ejection fraction. Identification and proper treatment institution are of paramount importance as they have >4 fold risk of death

---

[*] Corresponding Author: Lovely Chhabra, MD, 80 Seymour Street, Hartford, CT (06102),USA, Tel: +1-860-545-5000, Fax: +1-888-598-6647, Email: lovids@hotmail.com.

compared to the general population. Non cardiac factors have also been reported to increase the risk of diastolic dysfunction in patients with LVH. Atrial fibrillation is the most common supraventricular arrhythmia associated with LVH.

Value of clinical examination in the diagnosis of LVH in patients without any complications is limited. Though echocardiogram is one of the gold standard investigation, the inexpensive and easily available electrocardiogram (EKG) is the most commonly used modality. The most common abnormalities noticed in EKG are increased QRS voltage and duration, leftward axis, left atrial abnormality and repolarization abnormalities. Multiple criteria have been proposed for the diagnosis. The sensitivity and specificity depends on the criterion used. Studies have shown that use of multiple criteria has improved the diagnostic accuracy. Non-cardiac confounders have also been reported to affect the sensitivity and specificity of the criteria. Separate criteria for computer based interpretations have been proposed based on regression models. Apart from the diagnosis, EKG is also useful in prognostication. Regression of EKG changes of LVH with treatment of underlying factors, has been shown to correlate with reduction in risk for adverse cardiovascular outcomes. American Society of echocardiography has proposed guidelines for the diagnosis of LVH by echocardiogram.

Treatment of LVH is primarily targeted at the causative factors. Complete normalization of LVH has been shown in patients, who had the corrective measures for the mechanical problem causing the increased wall stress. However, this near normal reversal is not seen with treatment of hypertension. The degree of reversal has been shown to correlate with adequacy of control and also the agent used for therapy. Complications secondary to LVH should be managed based on the problems and attempts should be made to preserve sinus rhythm and avoid tachycardia for better outcomes. Regression of LVH with adequate treatment has been shown to decrease the cardiovascular risk significantly. In case of CKD, maintenance of hemoglobin between 10 to 12 grams/dl has shown reduction in left ventricular mass index and improved outcomes.

Introduction

Left Ventricular Hypertrophy (LVH) is defined as an increase in the mass of the left ventricle secondary to increase in wall thickness or increase in cavity size or both. LVH is not a disease per se and is usually a compensatory response by heart to hemodynamic overload. According to Laplace's Law,

Stress on any region of the myocardium = Pressure X Radius / 2 X Wall thickness.

Thus, increase in either of the variables in the numerator will necessitate increase in wall thickness to maintain the wall stress and indirectly the stroke volume [1]. Though alternate mechanisms like (1) use of Frank-Starling mechanism to increase cross bridge formation; and (2) recruit neuro-hormonal mechanisms to increase contractility compensate in the acute phase, both have limitations. Neuro-hormonal mechanisms can have deleterious effects when the insult persists chronically. Sustained pressure overload as in patients with aortic stenosis and hypertension sarcomeres are added in parallel resulting in increased mass to volume ratio (concentric hypertrophy). In volume overload state as in mitral or aortic regurgitation, the sarcomeres are added in series resulting in decreased mass to volume ratio (Eccentric Hypertrophy) [2]. Hypertrophic and infiltrative cardiomyopathies are distinct disorders secondary to genetic mutation. The pathogenesis is different and is not dealt with in this chapter.

Risk Factors

A number of conditions may predispose to the development of left ventricular hypertrophy. They can be classified based on the mechanism of induction of LVH:

1. Pressure Overload
   - Systemic hypertension
   - Aortic Stenosis
2. Volume Overload
   - Mitral Regurgitation
   - Aortic regurgitation
   - Anemia
   - Arterio-Venous Fistula.
3. Infiltrative disorders
   - Fabry's Disease
   - Hemochromatosis
   - Amyloidosis
4. Inherited
   - Hypertrophic obstructive cardiomyopathy

Among hypertensives, multiple independent variables have been shown to affect / predict LVH like exaggerated transient elevation in blood pressure (BP) during mental stress, daily BP load (% of pressure more than 135/85 during day and 120/80 during night), nocturnal hypertension and peak exercise blood pressure [3, 4]. This stresses the importance of guiding treatment to ambulatory BP recordings rather than to casual BP checks at the clinician's office. Studies have shown contradicting results about the role of gender towards development of LVH [5, 6]. Interestingly in a pooled analysis both eccentric and concentric pattern was noticed in hypertensive population, with eccentric morphology being most frequent [6].

Genetic factors have been shown to promote or retard the development of LVH, accounting for differences in the left ventricular mass between populations with similar degree of hypertension. DD genotype of the ACE gene [7], 9 bp deletion of the bradykinin receptor gene (B2BKR) [8] and overexpression of activated protein C [9] have shown to independently influence LVH. Hypertension with chronic kidney disease (CKD) in early stages causes a mixed pattern of LVH more frequently – increase in both diameter and thickness, with a trend towards concentric morphology with progression of worsening renal function [10]. Though multiple factors have been identified to contribute to LVH in patients with moderate kidney disease, systolic blood pressure and inflammatory marker C -reactive protein were the only independent predictors of left ventricular mass index [11]. Obesity is also an independent predictor of LVH. Obese people more frequently have eccentric rather than concentric morphology [12].

Prevalence

LVH prevalence depends on the criteria and modality used for diagnosis. Electrocardiograms and M-mode echocardiograms are the investigations used to diagnose LVH in the prevalence studies. Multiple criteria have been reported to be diagnostic of LVH in either of the modalities, the details of which will be discussed later. Based on the recent reviews, 24% of men and 16% of women hypertensives were reported to have LVH based on electrocardiograms [13]. Based on 2D Echocardiogram, LVH prevalence varied from 35.6% to 40.9% depending on the criteria (Conservative vs. less restrictive) used for diagnosis [6]. Interestingly, there was no gender difference identified in the prevalence based on the echocardiogram [6]. Very less isolated hypertensive patients with normal electrocardiogram have been shown to have mild LVH based on echocardiogram; however the percentage has not been statistically significant to warrant echocardiogram as the first line screening tool for LVH [14].

In patients with CKD, 47% prevalence was reported in pre-dialysis population [15]; 42% at the start of dialysis and 75% of patients who have been on dialysis for 10 years [16, 17]. 56% of obese population was also found to have LVH with an odds ratio of 4.19 compared to non-obese patients based on a pooled meta-analysis [12]. Though valvular heart disease has been associated with LVH, there is no reported prevalence. Earlier diagnosis, more intense follow up and early intervention in the current practice may have contributed to much less frequency of LVH associated with valvular heart disease.

Pathogenesis

Multiple theories and mediators have been proposed in the pathogenesis of left ventricular hypertrophy without direct evidence. In vivo, heart muscle within hours of pressure overload has shown increase in myosin heavy chain synthesis by 35% and this was believed to be secondary to translational efficiency [18]. However in case of volume overload, the increase in mass of left ventricle was thought be from decrease in myosin heavy chain degradation rate [19]. Complex changes in gene re-programming are usually associated with both forms of hypertrophy [20]. These changes include:

1. Re-expression of fetal cardiac genes including genes to modify motor unit composition and regulation, energy metabolism and encoding components of hormonal pathways.
2. Variable or late blunted response occurs in other genes that modify intracellular ion homeostasis like down regulation of sarcoplasmic reticulum calcium ATPase, up regulation of Na^+/Ca^{2+} exchanger.
3. Down regulation of key parasympathetic and sympathetic receptors.

Focal adhesion complex (FAC) has been hypothesized to act as transducer, transmitting the mechanical forces from stretch/ pressure into biochemical events [21]. FAC is the link between integrin's supporting the cytoskeleton of myocytes and the extracellular matrix (ECM). ECM also has many kinases implicated in the signaling process including tyrosine-phosphorylated kinases and serine-threonine kinases [22]. Disruption of cell-cell or cell-ECM contact has been shown to modulate the cell growth and apoptosis, but the exact sequence of events has not been elucidated [23].

This biomechanical transduction is usually also accompanied by recruitment of the G-protein coupled neuro-hormones (Angiotensin II and endothelin) and likely serves to amplify the growth signal triggered by the mechanical event [2]. Their exact role in the pathogenesis and amount of contribution to the clinical LVH is still unclear and studies have shown contradicting results. Other signaling molecule recently studied was the calcineurin, overexpression of which was associated with hypertrophic phenotype in animal models [24]. However calcineurin inhibitors failed to suppress experimental hypertrophy in animal models [25].

Apart from the myocytes growth, connective tissue architecture is also altered in patients with hypertrophy as evidenced by autopsy and biopsy studies. The complex collagen seen in the heart interlacing the myocytes translates individual myocyte force generation into a coordinated ventricular contraction [26]. The reactive fibrosis as noticed in pathological hypertrophies are characterized by both perivascular and interstitial fibrosis. Defective cell-ECM contact, myocardial ischemia or the local activation of trophic peptides have been proposed to be the likely triggers for the increase in collagen [2].

In volume overload state, the ECM remodeling follows a different pathophysiology as compared to the pressure overload state. The hypertrophy associated with volume overload state is due to combination of both myocyte elongation and changes in collagen cross-linking and weave [27, 28]. The changes in collagen primarily are increase in elasticity and muscle fiber slippage due to dissolution of the collagen weave enabling increase in chamber size[29]. Activated matrix metallo-proteinases (MMPs), a family of zinc containing proteins have been accounted for the dissolution based on observations in animal models and humans with end-stage dilated cardiomyopathies [30]. Examples of MMPs include collagenases, gelatinases and membrane type MMPs.

Clinical Implications

Though not a primary disease process, LVH can have varied clinical presentations and implications. Most of the people with LVH may remain in a compensated state for years before becoming symptomatic. Loss of exercise reserve is usually the first symptom/sign. The spectrum of manifestations may be due to physiological changes from LVH versus anatomical changes or a combination of both.

Diastolic Dysfunction

The dynamics of passive LV filling and the relationship between diastolic volume and pressure are influenced by the thickness of the wall and its composition, particularly collagen deposition and its architecture. The rate and magnitude of diastolic filling depends on the trans-mitral pressure gradient which in turn is dependent on both left atrial pressure and active fall of LV pressure to its nadir during relaxation [2]. In case of LVH, thick myocardium and altered collagen amount and deposition, leads to slow and incomplete relaxation causing diastolic dysfunction. Apart from the mechanical factors, down regulation of SERCA-2 (ATP dependent sarcoplasmic reticulum pumps) was shown to cause dysregulation of intracellular calcium and affect the rate of relaxation of myocardium in animal models. This in turn can affect the diastolic pressure volume relationship [2].

Diastolic dysfunction causes elevated end diastolic pressure and pressure/volume back in atrium secondary to incomplete passive emptying leading to heart failure. Three patterns of LV filling have been identified [31, 32]

1. Slowed relaxation – reduced early diastolic inflow velocity with a compensatory increase in filling due to atrial contraction (Decreased E/A ratio)
2. Pseudo-normalization – preserved ratio of contribution from early diastolic filling and atrial contraction, but a rapid deceleration of early mitral inflow (Preserved E/A/ ratio).
3. Restrictive pattern – all filling occurs explosively in early diastole with a very short deceleration time.

A case control series from Framingham heart study showed 51% of the subjects having heart failure had preserved ejection fraction [33]. As ventricular filling is very much dependent on the atrial contraction, atrial fibrillation is usually very poorly tolerated by patients with LVH and may provoke heart failure in a previously compensated patient[2].

Gender and age have impacts on the left ventricular hypertrophy. Elder population with comparable severities of aortic stenosis has been shown to have much severe hypertrophy, interstitial fibrosis and resultant impaired relaxation with elevated filling indices compared to younger population [34]. Men are more likely to have cavity enlargement and increased diastolic myocardial stiffness compared to women with similar disease [35]. Heart failure patients with normal ejection fraction have >4-fold mortality risk compared to general population [33]. Inability to augment LV volume secondary to stiffness and elevated filling pressures may severely limit exercise cardiac output and exercise reserve [2].

Arrhythmia

LVH is also an independent risk factor for sudden cardiac death (SCD) [36]. In patients with electrocardiographic pattern of LVH, six fold increased risk of sudden cardiac death among men and a threefold increase in women have been reported based on data from Framingham heart study [37]. On the contrary based on echocardiographic findings, each 50 g/m2 increase in left ventricular mass contributed to a relative risk of death from cardiovascular disease : 1.73 in men and 2.12 in women [38].

Among the supraventricular arrhythmias, atrial fibrillation is the most common arrhythmia associated with LVH. Based on Framingham heart study data, patients with LVH have 2 times more risk to develop atrial fibrillation [39]. Age and left ventricular mass are the independent predictors of developing atrial fibrillation [40]. A 3-fold increase of sudden cardiac death has also been reported in patients with LVH developing atrial fibrillation [41]. In small case series, premature supraventricular beats were found to be more frequent in patients with LVH [42].

Ventricular premature beats (VPB's) have also been consistently associated with LVH and for every 1 mm increase in wall thickness, two to three fold increase in the occurrence of

VPB's is noted [43]. Reduction in the sub-endocardial blood flow with resultant fibrosis/ scar seen in patients with LVH becomes the substrate for the VPB's and also malignant arrhythmia. Eccentric hypertrophy is associated with more severe arrhythmias than concentric hypertrophy [44]. Electrophysiological changes reported at the hypertrophied myocytes are lengthening of action potential duration and dispersion, slowing of membrane repolarization with resultant QT prolongation and generation of delayed after depolarization. These observations are from animal studies and these changes could contribute to the development of ventricular arrhythmias [45, 46, 47]. Interstitial fibrosis seen in patients with LVH facilitates the generated re-entry circuits [48]. T wave alternans; beat to beat variability in the timing and morphology of repolarization waves seen in patients with LVH has been associated with increased risk for sudden death [49].

Systolic Dysfunction

On the contrary to diastolic dysfunction in patients with LVH, the pathophysiology behind systolic dysfunction noticed in patients with long standing pressure / volume overload has not been clearly elucidated. Subendocardial ischemia seen in patients with LVH causing myocardial fibrosis is one postulated mechanism [50]. Dysregulation of calcium homeostasis and apoptosis causing loss of myocytes are other theories speculated to contribute to the impaired contractility noticed in patients with chronic hypertrophy [51, 52]. Clinically the presentation or manifestation would be loss of exercise capacity and heart failure.

Myocardial Ischemia

Framingham heart study showed that LVH, by itself is an independent risk factor for acute myocardial infarction. LVH has been attributed to increase the risk of developing overt coronary artery disease by 3 fold even after adjustments for hypertension [37]. Reduced density of capillaries and inability to vasodilate secondary to increase need or vasodilatory medications due to mechanical restriction from increased muscle mass may decrease the coronary reserve in patients with LVH and limit their exercise capacity [53]. Coronary occlusion has also been shown to have greater degree of infarction along with higher morbidity and mortality in patients with LVH [54].

Diagnosis

The predominant clinical examination finding in LVH is noticed at the apex beat, point of maximum impulse – the downward and lateral most point in the chest, where cardiac impulse can be maximum felt. The apex beat is more sustained in cases of LVH due to pressure overload state – concentric hypertrophy and displaced outward and downward in volume overload state – eccentric hypertrophy. As far as the diagnostic modalities for objective evidence, the electrocardiogram (EKG) and echocardiography are two important non-invasive tools used for diagnosing left ventricular hypertrophy (LVH). Though echocardiogram has always been the gold standard for diagnosis of LVH along with magnetic resonance imaging, electrocardiogram is the most commonly used modality secondary to its low cost and easy availability.

Left ventricular hypertrophy can have five major EKG findings: increased QRS voltage and duration in the precordial and limb leads, horizontal or left axis deviation ($\leq$ -30°), left atrial abnormality, and repolarization (ST-T) abnormalities [55, 56, 57]. Many of the EKG findings in LVH can be explained secondary to the increased left ventricular mass seen in this population. The QRS duration prolongation can be subtle or be evident as incomplete or complete left bundle branch block. The ST-T changes noted in LVH termed as 'LV strain pattern' are postulated to be secondary to primary repolarization abnormality of the hypertrophied myocardium or associated sub-endocardial ischemia.ST-T changes associated with LVH have been shown to correlate with presence of coronary artery disease and greater left ventricular mass [58].

Left atrial abnormality (LAA) is usually increased duration of P waves ($\geq$120 ms) in the limb leads and/or biphasic P waves with a prominent negative P-terminal force in V1 ($\geq$40 ms in duration and/or $\geq$1 mV in depth). LAA along with LBBB has been shown to have high sensitivity and specificity (80 and 89% respectively) in predicting LVH [59].

Electrocardiographic Criteria

Multiple criteria have been proposed for the diagnosis of LVH based on electrocardiography, as listed in table 1. The sensitivities and specificities of the criteria have been shown to vary between 20-60% and 80-100% respectively based on autopsy correlations [60]. False negatives and false positives are not uncommon especially in the setting of mild to moderate hypertrophy and underlying chronic obstructive lung disease. Specific cardiac conditions leading on to the LVH have also been shown to affect the sensitivity of various criteria in diagnosing LVH [61]. In general, electrocardiograms have improved sensitivity for LVH diagnosis in patients with systemic hypertension and valvular heart disease. QRS axis of less than -30 degrees was most often seen in patients with left ventricular hypertrophy and coronary artery disease [61]. On the contrary, presence of LVH has also been shown to significantly reduce the sensitivity of the electrocardiographic diagnostic dyad for emphysema (Combination of the frontal vertical P-Vector and narrow QRS duration), as it causes widening of the QRS duration [62].

Based on prospective epidemiological studies, various factors have been shown to affect the sensitivity of the EKG in diagnosing LVH. Female gender and smokers had marginally lower sensitivity than their counterparts [63]. Body mass index inversely correlated to sensitivity and sensitivity increased with age [63].

Criteria specific correlations of LVH diagnosis with autopsy findings have shown differential sensitivity and specificity for each, with Cornell criteria having high sensitivity (42%) among the group with preserved specificity (96%) [60]. Similarly, validity of the different criteria have been studied under different non-cardiac confounders. The sensitivity of Cornell voltage and duration criteria and Perugia score did not change in obese individuals compared to Sokolow-Lyon and Romhilt-Estes criteria [64]. Sokolow-Lyon criteria have lower specificity for diagnosis of LVH in African population compared to Caucasians [65].

In addition to the above clinical criteria, a regression criterion has been proposed for computer based interpretations. This criterion is based on regression models using electrocardiographic and demographic variables with independent predictive value for LVH [60]. There are separate equations for patients in sinus rhythm and atrial fibrillation (Table 2). This criterion was shown to improve sensitivity to 62% and maintain specificity (92%) based on correlation with autopsy findings [60].

Table 1. Criteria used for the diagnosis of LVH based on electrocardiography

	Name of the criteria	EKG findings
1.	Sokolow-Lyon index	SV1 + R in V5 or V6 > 3.5 mV and/or R aVL $\geq$1.1 mV (11 mm)
2.	Cornell voltage index	Male: RaVL + SV3 > 2.8mV (28mm) Female: RaVL + SV3 > 2.0mV (20mm)
3.	Cornell duration criteria	Male: (SV3+RaVL)×QRS duration > 2440 milliseconds Female: (SV3+(RaVL+8))×QRS duration > 2440 ms
4.	Perugia Score	Male: RaVL + SV3 > 2.4mV Female: RaVL + SV3 > 2.0mV

5.	Romhilt-Estes scores	Excessive amplitude - 3 points:
		    largest R or S wave in limb leads $\geq$ 20 mV or
		    S wave in V1 or V2 $\geq$ 30 mV or
		    R wave in V5 or V6 $\geq$ 30 mV.
		
		ST-T wave changes typical of LVH
		    Taking Digitalis – 1 point
		    Not Taking Digitalis – 3 point
		
		Left atrial abnormality
		P terminal force in V1 is 1 mm or more in depth with a duration 40ms - 3 points.
		
		Left axis deviation of more than (−30°) - 2 points.
		
		QRS duration $\geq$ 90ms – 1 point.
		
		Intrinsicoid deflection in V5 or V6 $\geq$0.05 s – 1 point.
		
		Score of 5 or more indicates "definite" LVH; a score of 4 indicates "probable" LVH.

Table 2. Multiple logistic regression exponents for detection of LVH [60]

For patients in normal sinus rhythm	Exponent = 4.558 − 0.092 x (RaVL + SV3) − 0.306 x TV1 − 0.212 x QRS − 0.278 x PTFV1 − 0.559 x Sex
For patients in atrial fibrillation	Exponent = 5.045 − 0.093 x (RaVL + SV3) − 0.312 x TV1 − 0.325 x QRS − 0.602 x Sex
Partition Value of exponent for detection of LVH	In Sinus Rhythm : LVH < -1.55 In Atrial Fibrillation : LVH < - 1.20
Units of Measurement: Voltages of RaVL, SV3 and TV1 in mm (1mm = 0.1 mV); QRS duration in seconds X 100; P terminal force in lead V1 (PTFV1) in mm x sec based on area; Sex entered as 1.0 for men and 2.0 for women.	

Total 12-lead QRS amplitude (>175 mm) was also proposed to predict LVH, especially in patients with aortic stenosis, aortic regurgitation and hypertrophic cardiomyopathy. It was also postulated to be more sensitive than the other criteria for diagnosis of LVH under above circumstances [66]. Later a refinement to the above criteria was suggested in view of redundancy noted from duplication of the output from limb leads. It was postulated that total QRS amplitude minus (R,L,F voltage) to be a better criterion, with > 110 mm cutoff serving as the most accurate index (best sensitivity, specificity, NPV and PPV) even in unselected patient population [67].

Usefulness and Limitations

Despite the multiple limitations in contribution towards diagnosis of LVH, electrocardiograms have role in prognostication. Hypertensive patients with electrocardiographic and echocardiographic evidence of LVH were found to have greater left ventricular mass than their counterparts with only echocardiographic evidence [68]. The mass is highest in those associated with strain pattern on electrocardiogram. Patients with EKG evidence of LVH have consistently been shown to have increased risk for major adverse cardiovascular events (MACE) like myocardial infarction, congestive heart failure and death from cardiovascular causes. The risk has been shown to correlate with the baseline voltage and accompanying repolarization abnormalities.

Serial EKG monitoring through the treatment period of the primary driving has been shown to predict outcomes. Patients with serial decline in voltage and repolarization abnormalities had reduction of the risk for MACE than those with no change. On the contrary, patients with increase in the above parameters on serial EKG while on treatment period had increased risk for MACE [69, 70]. This was consistently shown in subgroup analysis of multiple studies including HOPE trial [71] and Framingham heart study group. In a sub-study from LIFE trial, it was shown that similar strong correlation existed between changing left ventricular mass with cardiovascular morbidity and mortality [72]. However, careful attention should be paid to the confounding factors on follow up which can affect QRS voltage and mimic serial improvement. Examples of such factors include weight gain, anasarca, pleural effusion, pericardial effusion and increased severity of chronic obstructive pulmonary disease.

Echocardiography

In view of the low sensitivity of ECG in detecting LVH, echocardiography has become the preferred mode of investigation. In addition to the detection of LVH, echocardiographic examination can also permit quantification of left ventricular (LV) mass and give important information about the etiology of LVH (such as aortic or mitral valve disease, or hypertrophic cardiomyopathy), cardiac structure and functions, such as the degree of atrial enlargement, ventricular geometric pattern and diastolic dysfunction. The prevalence rates of LVH as assessed by echocardiography markedly varies among studies, ranging from 3 to 77%, depending on the clinical characteristics of the population studied and diagnostic criteria applied. Available data on LVH prevalence are mostly derived from population-based studies and selected hypertensive cohorts with rather scanty data available from surveys conducted in the clinical practice.

Echocardiographic Diagnosis of LVH

Most of the echocardiographic studies of left ventricular hypertrophy have relied on M-mode echocardiography. The diagnostic criteria include a left ventricular mass index $\geq$134 and $\geq$110 g/m2 body surface area in males and females, respectively. However, M-mode echocardiography has limitations in forms of a relatively low yield in older patients, suboptimal reproducibility, erroneous results in distorted ventricles, and use of a geometric algorithm overestimating the mass.

Two-dimensional echocardiography increase the precision and produce estimates of left ventricular mass that are similar to the values derived from pathology, magnetic resonance imaging, and computed tomography. The most commonly used two-dimensional method validated by the American Society of Echocardiography for measurement of left ventricular mass is area-length and truncated ellipse.

The recent guidelines published from the society for diagnosis of left ventricular hypertrophy included criteria for mild, moderate, and severe left ventricular hypertrophy for men as 103 to 116, 117 to 130, >130 g/m2 and for women as 89 to 100, 101 to 112, >112 g/m2, respectively. In terms of prognostic value, it is established that echocardiographically determined LVH is one of the powerful independent risk factors for cardiovascular morbidity, complications, and mortality.

Treatment

LVH management is primarily targeted at the causative factors and the complications. As LVH is a dynamic process, adequate therapies towards the driving factor may retard or even reverse the hypertrophy. There is evidence from previous studies to suggest a rapid reduction in myocyte hypertrophy and LV mass (approx. 35% reduction) within weeks of normalization of systolic load in patients with aortic stenosis by valve replacement [73]. It was also evident that there might be a transient elevation in the fraction of the collagen in the initial phase as the myocytes regress rapidly compared to collagen, however with sustained reduction of systolic load, the collagen content also regresses reverting to near normal left ventricular wall thickness and diastolic parameters [73].

Unlike the mechanical valvular disorders, control of hypertension was not consistently associated with reversal of hypertrophy to near normal state [74]. This could be secondary to inadequate control of blood pressures versus unaddressed neuro-hormonal mechanisms causing left ventricular hypertrophy sharing pathophysiology with hypertension. This partially explains the differential response of left ventricular hypertrophy to the agents used in treatment of hypertension. Multiple studies have been conducted comparing head to head efficacy of different medications on LVH regression for example PRESERVE [75] trial comparing Enalapril with Nifedipine; and LIFE [76] comparing Losartan with Atenolol. Based on a meta-analysis [77], the relative reduction of left ventricular hypertrophy among various antihypertensive agents were:

1. Angiotensin II receptor blockers – 13 percent
2. Calcium channel blockers – 11 percent
3. Angiotensin converting enzyme inhibitors – 10 percent
4. Diuretics – 8 percent
5. Beta blockers – 6 percent

In a small double blind trial, Losartan was shown to attenuate the progression of myocardial hypertrophy and fibrosis in patients with LVH independent of its effect on blood pressure control [78].

Management of complications of LVH like heart failure and VPB's are primarily targeted at the specific complication like fluid management for heart failure, along with continued efforts to correct the primary causative factor for LVH. Regression of LVH appears to be associated with reduction in ventricular arrhythmias based on animal studies and also observations in humans [46, 79]. Similarly, normalization of LVH changes in electrocardiogram while being on treatment was associated with significant reduction in sudden cardiac death [80]. In case of atrial fibrillation associated with LVH, attempts should be made to preserve sinus rhythm and avoid tachycardia as left ventricular filling is dependent on the contribution from the atrial contraction [2]. Regression of electrocardiographic LVH with appropriate therapy was associated with reduced incidence of new onset atrial fibrillation independent of blood pressure reduction and treatment modality used [81].

In case of LVH associated with CKD and anemia, improving anemia with use of epoetin to targeted hemoglobin goal between 10 – 12 g/dl showed significant reduction in left ventricular mass index. However target hemoglobin of > 12 did not show any sustained improvement rate [82] Management of LVH secondary to infiltrative disorders should again be directed at the primary disorder. In case of HOCM, treatment strategy would be to relieve the obstruction at the left ventricular outflow tract either medically or surgically. The details of the treatment options for HOCM and infiltrative disorders are not covered in this chapter.

References

[1]   Gunther S, Grossman W. Determinants of ventricular function in pressure-overload hypertrophy in man. *Circulation*. 1979 Apr;59(4):679-88.
[2]   Lorell BH, Carabello BA. Left ventricular hypertrophy: pathogenesis, detection, and prognosis. *Circulation*. 2000 Jul 25;102(4):470-9.
[3]   Schnall PL, Pieper C, Schwartz JE, et al. The relationship between 'job strain,' workplace diastolic blood pressure, and left ventricular mass index. Results of a case-control study. *JAMA*. 1990 Apr 11; 263(14):1929-35.
[4]   Devereux RB, Pickering TG, Harshfield GA, et al. Left ventricular hypertrophy in patients with hypertension: importance of blood pressure response to regularly recurring stress. *Circulation*. 1983 Sep;68(3):470-6.
[5]   Schirmer H, Lunde P, Rasmussen K. Prevalence of left ventricular hypertrophy in a general population; The Tromsø Study. *Eur. Heart J*. 1999 Mar;20(6):429-38.

[6]   Cuspidi C, Sala C, Negri F, Mancia G, Morganti A. Prevalence of left-ventricular hypertrophy in hypertension: an updated review of echocardiographic studies. *J. Hum. Hypertens.* 2012 Jun;26(6):343-9.

[7]   Schunkert H, Hense HW, Holmer SR, et al. Association between a deletion polymorphism of the angiotensin-converting-enzyme gene and left ventricular hypertrophy. *N. Engl. J. Med.* 1994 Jun 9;330(23):1634-8.

[8]   Brull D, Dhamrait S, Myerson S, et al. Bradykinin B2BKR receptor polymorphism and left-ventricular growth response. *Lancet.* 2001 Oct 6;358(9288):1155-6.

[9]   Bowman JC, Steinberg SF, Jiang T, et al. Expression of protein kinase C beta in the heart causes hypertrophy in adult mice and sudden death in neonates. *J. Clin. Invest.* 1997 Nov 1;100(9):2189-95.

[10]   Nardi E, Palermo A, Mulè G, et al.Left ventricular hypertrophy and geometry in hypertensive patients with chronic kidney disease. *J. Hypertens.* 2009 Mar;27(3):633-41.

[11]   Cottone S, Nardi E, Mulè G, et al. Association between biomarkers of inflammation and left ventricular hypertrophy in moderate chronic kidney disease. *Clin. Nephrol.* 2007 Apr;67(4):209-16.

[12]   Cuspidi C, Rescaldani M, Sala C, Grassi G. Left-ventricular hypertrophy and obesity: a systematic review and meta-analysis of echocardiographic studies. *J. Hypertens.* 2014 Jan;32(1):16-25.

[13]   Cuspidi C, Rescaldani M, Sala C, et al. Prevalence of electrocardiographic left ventricular hypertrophy in human hypertension: an updated review. *J. Hypertens.* 2012 Nov;30(11):2066-73.

[14]   Nardi E, Palermo A, Mulè G, et al. Prevalence and predictors of left ventricular hypertrophy in patients with hypertension and normal electrocardiogram. *Eur. J. Prev. Cardiol.* 2013 Oct;20(5):854-61.

[15]   Levin A, Singer J, Thompson CR, Ross H, Lewis M. Prevalent left ventricular hypertrophy in the predialysis population: identifying opportunities for intervention. *Am. J. Kidney Dis.* 1996 Mar;27(3):347-54.

[16]   Parfrey PS, Foley RN, Harnett JD, et al. Outcome and risk factors for left ventricular disorders in chronic uraemia. *Nephrol. Dial. Transplant.* 1996 Jul;11(7):1277-85.

[17]   Parfrey PS, Foley RN. The clinical epidemiology of cardiac disease in chronic renal failure. *J. Am. Soc. Nephrol.* 1999 Jul;10(7):1606-15.

[18]   Imamura T, McDermott PJ, Kent RL, et al. Acute changes in myosin heavy chain synthesis rate in pressure versus volume overload. *Circ. Res.* 1994 Sep;75(3):418-25.

[19]   Matsuo T, Carabello BA, Nagatomo Y, et al. Mechanisms of cardiac hypertrophy in canine volume overload. . *Am. J. Physiol.* 1998 Jul;275(1 Pt 2):H65-74.

[20]   Swynghedauw B. Molecular mechanisms of myocardial remodeling. *Physiol. Rev.* 1999; 79: 216-261.

[21]   Borg TK, Burgess ML. Holding it all together: organization and functions of the extracellular matrix of the heart. *Heart Failure.* 1993; 8: 230-238.

[22]   Kuppuswamy D, Kerr C, Narishige T, et al. Association of tyrosine-phosphorylated c-Src with the cytoskeleton of hypertrophying myocardium. *J. Biol. Chem.* 1997 Feb 14;272(7):4500-8.

[23] McGill G, Shimamura A, Bates RC, et al. Loss of matrix adhesion triggers rapid transformation-selective apoptosis in fibroblasts. *J. Cell. Biol.* 1997 Aug 25;138(4): 901-11.

[24] Molkentin JD, Lu JR, Antos CL, et al. A calcineurin-dependent transcriptional pathway for cardiac hypertrophy. *Cell.* 1998 Apr 17;93(2):215-28.

[25] Zhang W, Kowal RC, Rusnak F, et al. Failure of calcineurin inhibitors to prevent pressure-overload left ventricular hypertrophy in rats. *Circ. Res.* 1999 Apr 2;84(6):722-8.

[26] Weber KT, Sun Y, Tyagi SC, et al. Collagen network of the myocardium: function, structural remodeling and regulatory mechanisms. *J. Mol. Cell. Cardiol.* 1994 Mar;26(3):279-92.

[27] Spinale FG, Ishihra K, Zile M, et al. Structural basis for changes in left ventricular function and geometry because of chronic mitral regurgitation and after correction of volume overload. *J. Thorac. Cardiovasc. Surg.* 1993 Dec;106(6):1147-57.

[28] Olivetti G, Capasso JM, Sonnenblick EH, et al.Side-to-side slippage of myocytes participates in ventricular wall remodeling acutely after myocardial infarction in rats. *Circ. Res.* 1990 Jul;67(1):23-34.

[29] Kato S, Spinale FG, Tanaka R, et al. Inhibition of collagen cross-linking: effects on fibrillar collagen and ventricular diastolic function. *Am. J. Physiol.* 1995 Sep;269(3 Pt 2):H863-8.

[30] Woessner JF Jr. Matrix metalloproteinases and their inhibitors in connective tissue remodeling. *FASEB J.* 1991 May;5(8):2145-54.

[31] Little WC, Downes TR. Clinical evaluation of left ventricular diastolic performance. *Prog. Cardiovasc. Dis.* 1990 Jan-Feb;32(4):273-90.

[32] Cohen GI, Pietrolungo JF, Thomas JD, et al. A practical guide to assessment of ventricular diastolic function using Doppler echocardiography. *J. Am. Coll. Cardiol.* 1996 Jun;27(7):1753-60.

[33] Vasan RS, Larson MG, Benjamin EJ, et al. Congestive heart failure in subjects with normal versus reduced left ventricular ejection fraction: prevalence and mortality in a population-based cohort. *J. Am. Coll. Cardiol.* 1999 Jun;33(7):1948-55.

[34] Villari B, Vassalli G, Schneider J, et al. Age dependency of left ventricular diastolic function in pressure overload hypertrophy. *J. Am. Coll. Cardiol.* 1997 Jan;29(1):181-6.

[35] Villari B, Campbell SE, Schneider J, et al. Sex-dependent differences in left ventricular function and structure in chronic pressure overload. *Eur. Heart J.* 1995 Oct;16(10):1410-9.

[36] Kannel WB, Doyle JT, McNamara PM, et al. Precursors of sudden coronary death. Factors related to the incidence of sudden death. *Circulation.* 1975 Apr;51(4):606-13.

[37] Kannel WB, Gordon T, Castelli WP, et al. Electrocardiographic left ventricular hypertrophy and risk of coronary heart disease. The Framingham study. *Ann. Intern. Med.* 1970 Jun;72(6):813-22.

[38] Koren MJ, Devereux RB, Casale PN, et al. Relation of left ventricular mass and geometry to morbidity and mortality in uncomplicated essential hypertension. *Ann. Intern. Med.* 1991 Mar 1;114(5):345-52.

[39] Kannel WB, Abbott RD, Savage DD, et al. Epidemiologic features of chronic atrial fibrillation: the Framingham study. *N. Engl. J. Med.* 1982 Apr 29;306(17):1018-22.

[40] Verdecchia P, Reboldi G, Gattobigio R, et al. Atrial fibrillation in hypertension: predictors and outcome. *Hypertension.* 2003 Feb;41(2):218-23.

[41] Okin PM, Bang CN, Wachtell K, et al. Relationship of sudden cardiac death to new-onset atrial fibrillation in hypertensive patients with left ventricular hypertrophy. *Circ. Arrhythm. Electrophysiol.* 2013 Apr;6(2):243-51.

[42] Melina D, Colivicchi F, Guerrera G, et al. Prevalence of left ventricular hypertrophy and cardiac arrhythmias in borderline hypertension. *Am. J. Hypertens.* 1992 Aug;5(8):570-3.

[43] Ghali JK, Kadakia S, Cooper RS, et al.Impact of left ventricular hypertrophy on ventricular arrhythmias in the absence of coronary artery disease. *J. Am. Coll. Cardiol.* 1991 May;17(6):1277-82.

[44] Levy D, Anderson KM, Plehn J, et al. Echocardiographically determined left ventricular structural and functional correlates of complex or frequent ventricular arrhythmias on one-hour ambulatory electrocardiographic monitoring. *Am. J. Cardiol.* 1987 Apr 1;59(8):836-40.

[45] Gillis AM, Mathison HJ, Kulisz E, et al. Dispersion of ventricular repolarization and ventricular fibrillation in left ventricular hypertrophy: influence of selective potassium channel blockers. *J. Pharmacol. Exp. Ther.* 2000 Jan;292(1):381-6.

[46] Rials SJ, Wu Y, Ford N, et al.Effect of left ventricular hypertrophy and its regression on ventricular electrophysiology and vulnerability to inducible arrhythmia in the feline heart. *Circulation.* 1995 Jan 15;91(2):426-30.

[47] Ben-David J, Zipes DP, Ayers GM, et al. Canine left ventricular hypertrophy predisposes to ventricular tachycardia induction by phase 2 early afterdepolarizations after administration of BAY K 8644. *J. Am. Coll. Cardiol.* 1992 Dec;20(7):1576-84.

[48] Mammarella A, Paradiso M, Basili S, et al. Morphologic left ventricular patterns and prevalence of high-grade ventricular arrhythmias in the normotensive and hypertensive elderly. *Adv. Ther.* 2000 Sep-Oct;17(5):222-9.

[49] Hennersdorf MG, Niebch V, Perings C, et al. T wave alternans and ventricular arrhythmias in arterial hypertension. *Hypertension.* 2001 Feb;37(2):199-203.

[50] Nakano K, Corin WJ, Spann JF Jr, et al. Abnormal subendocardial blood flow in pressure overload hypertrophy is associated with pacing-induced subendocardial dysfunction. *Circ. Res.* 1989 Dec;65(6):1555-64.

[51] Schlotthauer K, Schattmann J, Bers DM, et al. Frequency-dependent changes in contribution of SR Ca2+ to Ca2+ transients in failing human myocardium assessed with ryanodine. *J. Mol. Cell. Cardiol.* 1998 Jul;30(7):1285-94.

[52] Hamet P, Richard L, Dam TV, et al. Apoptosis in target organs of hypertension. *Hypertension.* 1995 Oct;26(4):642-8.

[53] Beache GM, Herzka DA, Boxerman JL, et al. Attenuated myocardial vasodilator response in patients with hypertensive hypertrophy revealed by oxygenation-dependent magnetic resonance imaging. *Circulation.* 2001 Sep 11;104(11):1214-7.

[54] Carluccio E, Tommasi S, Bentivoglio M, et al. Prognostic value of left ventricular hypertrophy and geometry in patients with a first, uncomplicated myocardial infarction. *Int. J. Cardiol.* 2000 Jul 31;74(2-3):177-83.

[55] Goldberger AL, Goldberger ZD, Shvilkin A. Goldberger's Clinical Electrocardiography: A Simplified Approach, 8th ed, Elsevier/Saunders, Philadelphia 2013.

[56] Mirvis, DM.. Electrocardiography: A Physiologic Approach, Mosby, St. Louis 1993.

[57] Mirvis, DM, Goldberger, AL. Electrocardiography. In: Braunwald's Heart Disease: A Textbook of Cardiovascular Medicine, 9th ed, Bonow, RO, Mann, DL, Zipes, DP, Libby, P (Eds), W.B. Saunders, Philadelphia 2011.

[58] Okin PM, Devereux RB, Nieminen MS, et al. Relationship of the electrocardiographic strain pattern to left ventricular structure and function in hypertensive patients: the LIFE study. Losartan Intervention for End point. *J. Am. Coll. Cardiol.* 2001 Aug;38(2):514-20.

[59] Mehta A, Jain AC, Mehta MC, et al. Usefulness of left atrial abnormality for predicting left ventricular hypertrophy in the presence of left bundle branch block. *Am. J. Cardiol.* 2000 Feb 1;85(3):354-9.

[60] Casale PN, Devereux RB, Alonso DR, et al. Improved sex-specific criteria of left ventricular hypertrophy for clinical and computer interpretation of electrocardiograms: validation with autopsy findings. *Circulation.* 1987 Mar;75(3):565-72.

[61] Murphy ML, Thenabadu PN, de Soyza N, et al. Sensitivity of electrocardiographic criteria for left ventricular hypertrophy according to type of cardiac disease. *Am. J. Cardiol.* 1985 Feb 15;55(5):545-9.

[62] Lanjewar SS, Chhabra L, Chaubey VK, et al. Diagnostic electrocardiographic dyad criteria of emphysema in left ventricular hypertrophy. . *Int. J. Chron. Obstruct. Pulmon. Dis.* 2013;8:591-4.

[63] Levy D, Labib SB, Anderson KM, et al. Determinants of sensitivity and specificity of electrocardiographic criteria for left ventricular hypertrophy. *Circulation.* 1990 Mar;81(3):815-20.

[64] da Costa W, Riera AR, Costa Fde A, et al. Correlation of electrocardiographic left ventricular hypertrophy criteria with left ventricular mass by echocardiogram in obese hypertensive patients. *J. Electrocardiol.* 2008 Nov-Dec;41(6):724-9.

[65] Vanezis AP, Bhopal R. Validity of electrocardiographic classification of left ventricular hypertrophy across adult ethnic groups with echocardiography as a standard. *J. Electrocardiol.* 2008 Sep-Oct;41(5):404-12.

[66] Dollar AL, Roberts WC. Usefulness of total 12-lead QRS voltage compared with other criteria for determining left ventricular hypertrophy in hypertrophic cardiomyopathy: analysis of 57 patients studied at necropsy. *Am. J. Med.* 1989 Oct;87(4):377-81.

[67] Kumar D, Bajaj R, Chhabra L, Spodick DH. Refinement of total 12-lead QRS voltage criteria for diagnosing left ventricular hypertrophy. *World journal of Cardiovascular disease*, 2013; (3) : 210-214.

[68] Fragola PV, Colivicchi F, Fabrizi E, et al. Assessment of left ventricular hypertrophy in patients with essential hypertension. A rational basis for the electrocardiogram. *Am. J. Hypertens.* 1993 Feb;6(2):164-9.

[69] Okin PM, Devereux RB, Jern S, et al. Regression of electrocardiographic left ventricular hypertrophy during antihypertensive treatment and the prediction of major cardiovascular events. *JAMA.*2004 Nov 17;292(19):2343-9.

[70] Levy D, Salomon M, D'Agostino RB, et al. Prognostic implications of baseline electrocardiographic features and their serial changes in subjects with left ventricular hypertrophy. *Circulation.* 1994 Oct;90(4):1786-93.

[71] Mathew J, Sleight P, Lonn E, et al. Reduction of cardiovascular risk by regression of electrocardiographic markers of left ventricular hypertrophy by the angiotensin-converting enzyme inhibitor ramipril. *Circulation.* 2001 Oct 2;104(14):1615-21.

[72] Devereux RB, Wachtell K, Gerdts E, et al. Prognostic significance of left ventricular mass change during treatment of hypertension. *JAMA.* 2004 Nov 17;292(19):2350-6.

[73] Villari B, Vassalli G, Monrad ES, et al. Normalization of diastolic dysfunction in aortic stenosis late after valve replacement. *Circulation.* 1995 May 1;91(9):2353-8.

[74] Dahlöf B, Pennert K, Hansson L. Reversal of left ventricular hypertrophy in hypertensive patients. A metaanalysis of 109 treatment studies. *Am. J. Hypertens.* 1992 Feb;5(2):95-110.

[75] Devereux RB, Palmieri V, Sharpe N, et al. Effects of once-daily angiotensin-converting enzyme inhibition and calcium channel blockade-based antihypertensive treatment regimens on left ventricular hypertrophy and diastolic filling in hypertension: the prospective randomized enalapril study evaluating regression of ventricular enlargement (preserve) trial. *Circulation.* 2001 Sep 11;104(11):1248-54.

[76] Okin PM, Devereux RB, Gerdts E, et al. Impact of diabetes mellitus on regression of electrocardiographic left ventricular hypertrophy and the prediction of outcome during antihypertensive therapy: the Losartan Intervention For Endpoint (LIFE) Reduction in Hypertension Study. *Circulation.* 2006 Mar 28;113(12):1588-96.

[77] Klingbeil AU, Schneider M, Martus P, et al. A meta-analysis of the effects of treatment on left ventricular mass in essential hypertension. *Am. J. Med.* 2003 Jul;115(1):41-6.

[78] Shimada YJ, Passeri JJ, Baggish AL, et al. Effects of losartan on left ventricular hypertrophy and fibrosis in patients with nonobstructive hypertrophic cardiomyopathy. *JACC Heart Fail.* 2013 Dec;1(6):480-7.

[79] Rials SJ, Wu Y, Xu X, et al. Regression of left ventricular hypertrophy with captopril restores normal ventricular action potential duration, dispersion of refractoriness, and vulnerability to inducible ventricular fibrillation. *Circulation.* 1997 Aug 19;96(4): 1330-6.

[80] Wachtell K, Okin PM, Olsen MH, et al. Regression of electrocardiographic left ventricular hypertrophy during antihypertensive therapy and reduction in sudden cardiac death: the LIFE Study. *Circulation.* 2007 Aug 14;116(7):700-5.

[81] Okin PM, Wachtell K, Devereux RB, et al. Regression of electrocardiographic left ventricular hypertrophy and decreased incidence of new-onset atrial fibrillation in patients with hypertension. *JAMA.* 2006 Sep 13;296(10):1242-8.

[82] Parfrey PS, Lauve M, Latremouille-Viau D, et al. Erythropoietin therapy and left ventricular mass index in CKD and ESRD patients: a meta-analysis. *Clin. J. Am. Soc. Nephrol.* 2009 Apr;4(4):755-62.

Chapter 2

Left Ventricular Hypertrophy, Fibrosis and Decompensation in Patients with Aortic Stenosis

Vassilis Vassiliou [1,2,*], *Calvin W. L. Chin* [3,4], *Tamir Malley* [1], *David E. Newby* [3], *Marc R. Dweck* [3,†] *and Sanjay K. Prasad* [1,2,†]

[1]Department of Cardiology and Cardiovascular Biomedical Research Unit,
Royal Brompton Hospital, London, UK
[2]National Heart and Lung Institute, Imperial College London, UK
[3]British Heart Foundation/ University Centre for Cardiovascular Science,
University of Edinburgh, UK
[4]Department of Cardiovascular Medicine,
National Heart Center Singapore, Singapore

Abstract

Aortic valve stenosis is the most common valvular heart disease in the Western world. It currently affects more than 7% of the population over the age of 60, with severe stenosis affecting in excess of 3% of people over the age of 75. In parallel with an aging population, the prevalence of aortic stenosis and need for surgery are expected to double over the next 20 years increasing further the burden on healthcare resources.

Left untreated aortic stenosis leads to an abnormally high pressure load on the left ventricle, a pathological process that induces myocyte hypertrophy and fibrosis. Initially, the adaptive process of increased wall thickness maintains normal wall stress, contraction and cardiac output. However, ultimately this becomes maladaptive leading to ventricular stiffness, an increase in myocyte hypertrophy and myocardial fibrosis eventually causing diastolic and systolic dysfunction and increased morbidity and mortality.

At present there is no effective medical therapy capable of altering this course and aortic valve intervention, usually in the form of surgical aortic valve replacement, is

[*] Corresponding author: Dr. Vassilis Vassiliou, Email: Vassiliou@doctors.org.uk.
[†] Joint Senior Authors

recommended by international guidelines in patients with severe stenosis and evidence of LV decompensation (either on the basis of symptoms or a reduced ejection fraction). Following aortic valve intervention patients demonstrate a variable degree of regression of the ventricular hypertrophy with favorable prognosis demonstrated in the cohort of patients with the highest level of regression.

In this chapter we will discuss the prevalence and mechanism of left ventricular hypertrophy, fibrosis and decompensation in patients with aortic stenosis. Through case examples we will illustrate common cases of patients with hypertrophy relating to AS and analyze the most recent guidelines from the American Heart Association/American College of Cardiology (2014) and European Society of Cardiology (2012) on managing patients with aortic stenosis.

Introduction

Aortic stenosis (AS) is the most common valvular heart disease in the Western world and is characterized by a progressive narrowing (or stenosis) of the aortic valve. Severe AS currently affects 3% of the population over the age of 75 [1] and in parallel with an aging population the prevalence of AS is expected to double over the next 20 years [2]. Currently, AS is the most common condition necessitating valve replacement surgery in the Western world, significantly contributing to increased morbidity, mortality and use of health resources [3].

If left untreated, AS leads to an abnormally high pressure load on the left ventricle (LV). This is a pathologic process- the ventricle initially responds appropriately with myocyte hypertrophy, followed by an increase in the LV wall thickness and mass. The increased thickness initially maintains normal wall stress and contraction according to La Place Law allowing normal wall contractility and normal cardiac output [4]. However ultimately this process becomes maladaptive, leading to ventricular stiffness, an increase in myocyte hypertrophy and myocardial fibrosis, eventually causing diastolic and systolic dysfunction and increased morbidity and mortality [5]. There is also significant variation in both the degree and pattern of hypertrophy and fibrosis observed in patients with AS, as a response to the pressure overload, with some patients with only moderate AS having a significant hypertrophic response while others with severe AS demonstrating normal wall thickness and mass. Ultimately, and usually following a significant hypertrophic response the LV will decompensate and fail unless the stenosis is relieved and the pressure load reduced [6, 7].

Left Ventricular Hypertrophy in Aortic Stenosis

When the LV is in a state of pressure overload, like in the case of AS, the wall stress increases according to the La Place Law. This suggests that the wall stress (T) is directly proportional to the pressure (P) according to the following equation, where r is the radius of the LV and h is the myocardial thickness.

$$T = (P \times r) / (2 \times h)$$

As a response to the increased pressure overload and in order to avoid the consequences of high stress on the wall, the myocardium's initial mechanism of adaptation is to increase myocyte size, wall thickness and mass, thus counterbalancing the high wall stress and maintaining cardiac output [8]. Given that the denominator of this equation is the wall thickness multiplied by a factor of two, even a small increase in the myocardial wall can lead to a significant decrease in the wall stress, allowing preservation of the LV systolic function and cardiac output.

A better understanding of the different patterns of LV remodeling and hypertrophy in aortic stenosis has been provided by Cardiovascular Magnetic Resonance (CMR) [9]. There are five pathological patterns of LV mass characterization, depending on the degree and site of hypertrophic changes as shown in Figure 1. A significant distinction in this classification relates to the use of the terms "hypertrophy" and "remodeling" when describing these changes. Hypertrophy specifically relates to an increased LV mass index (the LV mass indexed to the body surface area) when compared to healthy age and sex matched controls. Most commonly this is due to increased wall thickness but can occur in subjects with normal wall thickness if the left ventricle is dilated (e.g., in LV decompensation).

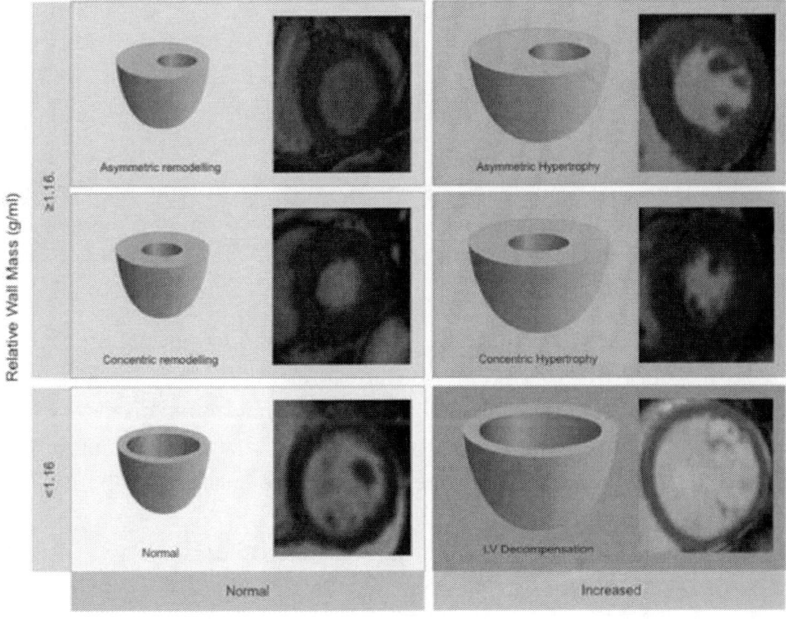

Figure 1. CMR characterized patterns of response to AS. Figure 1A (bottom left) represents normal ventricular structure with normal indexed LV mass and LV End Diastolic Volume (LVEDV) and a normal LV mass/volume (M/V) ratio. Figure 1B (middle left) represents concentric remodeling with normal overall LV mass but high LV M/V ratio. Figure 1C (top left) represents asymmetric remodeling with normal LV mass but high LV M/V ratio and evidence of asymmetric remodeling (rather than concentric hypertrophy) distinguishing it form 1B. Figure 1D (top right) represents asymmetric hypertrophy with increased overall LV mass index and increased M/V. Figure 1E (middle right) shows overall increased LV mass index and increased M/V but with absence of asymmetric hypertrophy, thus representing concentric hypertrophy and finally late in the transition process is figure 1F (bottom right) representing a dilated and decompensated LV with high overall LV mass due to the dilation and normal M/V ratio. Reproduced with permission from Dweck et al. [9].

Increased wall thickness can also occur in the context of a normal indexed mass, usually because the indexed LV End Diastolic Volume (LVEDV) is decreased, and is referred to as LV remodeling. Both LV remodeling and hypertrophy can be further subdivided into those with symmetrical wall thickening (concentric) and those with asymmetrical thickening usually observed in the septum (asymmetric) (Figure 2).

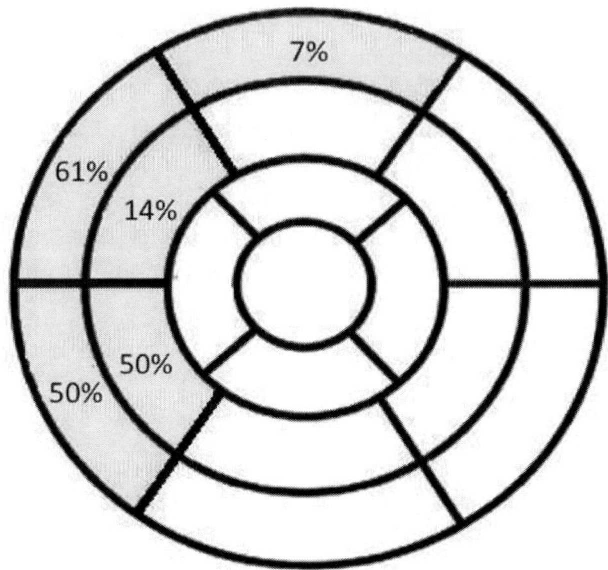

Figure 2. 17-segment model of the LV identifying the sites of maximal wall thickness in asymmetric remodeling and hypertrophy using CMR. This was predominantly seen at the septum. Reproduced with permission from Dweck et al. [9].

How patients transition between these different patterns of remodeling and hypertrophy remains unclear. However with prolonged exposure to an increased afterload ultimately the hypertrophic response of the left ventricle will decompensate, characterized by dilatation and reduced systolic function. This pattern is associated with an adverse outcome and worse peri-operative outcomes so that ideally surgery should be performed before this stage is reached.

Multiple studies have shown that only a weak correlation exists between the severity of AS and the degree of LV hypertrophy that develops. Indeed 10-20% of patients with severe AS have no LV hypertrophy [7, 10]. Sex related differences could partly explain this with women having smaller ventricles and lower mass [11]. This could potentially also relate to the relative estrogen and testosterone levels with the former protecting the myocardium from hypertrophy and the latter promoting it [12]. Other factors affecting hypertrophy include the metabolic syndrome, obesity, blood pressure control, and genetic factors such as the Angiotensin Converting Enzyme (ACE) I/D polymorphism [13] or even concomitant use of (ACE) inhibitors or beta blockers. This difference in hypertrophic response could partly explain why patients with similar degrees of valve obstruction often have very different degrees of symptom severity. Indeed it has been established that patients with a more advanced hypertrophic response have an adverse prognosis in AS [14] independent of valve stenosis severity, mirroring the findings in hypertensive heart disease [15].

In addition to hypertrophy, using CMR and following administration of a paramagnetic agent (e.g., gadolinium) one can accurately identify fibrosis (or "scarring") of the heart muscle [16, 17]. The transition from hypertrophy to heart failure is believed to be driven by a combination of myocyte cell death and progressive myocardial fibrosis [18]. The non-invasive detection of myocardial fibrosis in AS therefore holds potential as an objective means of detecting LV decompensation, indeed its presence has been closely linked to an advanced hypertrophic response and other markers of LV decompensation. In particular the association between fibrosis, hypertrophy, symptom development and adverse cardiovascular events in AS merits further discussion.

Myocardial Fibrosis in AS

In patients with AS the rate of progression from the asymptomatic state to developing symptoms of heart failure cannot be fully explained by valve hemodynamics alone and the role of hypertrophy in symptom development is gradually being appreciated. In addition to hypertrophy, myocardial fibrosis also appears to be implicated in the transition to this decompensated phase [9]. In the hypertrophic myocardium perfusion decreases and the systolic wall stress increases leading initially to interstitial fibrosis followed by replacement fibrosis [19].

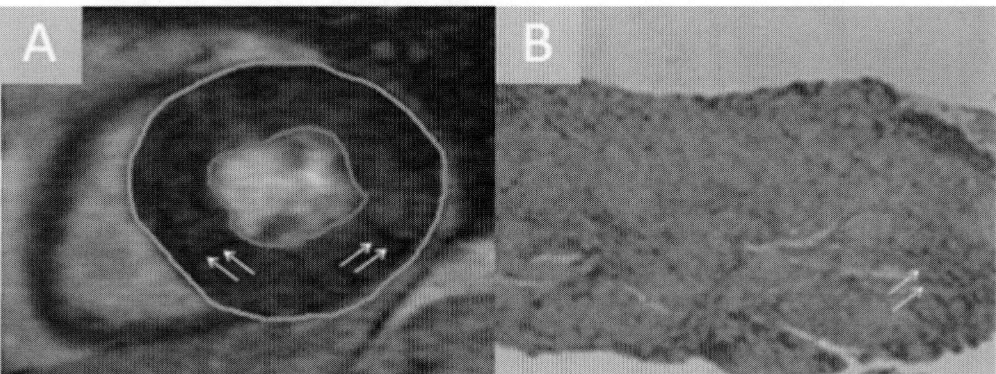

Figure 3. Image on the left (1A) demonstrating a CMR scan of the LV wall (included between the outside orange and inside green circles). The white arrows pointing at areas of enhancement after gadolinium administration indicative of fibrosis, or "scarring" of the myocardium. Figure 1B is a histological sample stained with picrosirius red confirming the presence of replacement fibrosis (white arrows) corresponding to the areas of the myocardium with enhancement seen at the CMR.

Histopathological studies have demonstrated that areas of fibrosis localize near areas of myocyte apoptosis and confirmed that fibrosis is an integral part of the hypertrophic process [2, 20]. Hein established that the transition point from myocardial hypertrophy to failure and initiation of symptoms is associated with increased myocyte apoptosis and fibrosis leading to the suggestion that myocardial fibrosis occurs as a form of scarring after myocyte injury and death [18].

Current guidelines determining the optimal timing for surgery are heavily dependent on the presence of symptoms or a substantial decline in LV ejection fraction [21, 22], both of which represent late features in the decompensation process in patients with AS and markers of potentially irreversible deterioration. As suggested by Dweck [2] and demonstrated in Figure 4, the development of symptoms or signs of systolic impairment usually follow myocardial hypertrophy and fibrosis. The optimal window for aortic valve replacement can be missed if we rely on the development of symptoms or existing signs of decompensation. There is therefore considerable interest in identifying earlier and more objective biomarkers of LV decompensation in aortic stenosis, with the detection of myocardial fibrosis in particular holding real promise.

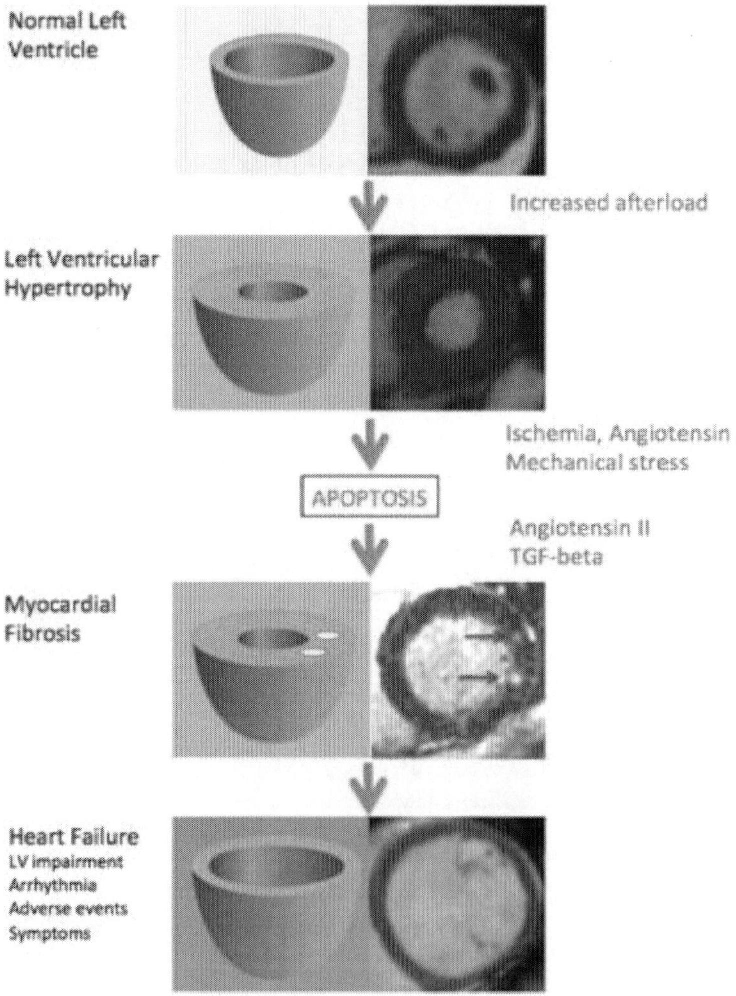

Figure 4. In patients with AS, due to increased afterload an initial adaptive hypertrophic response is seen restoring wall stress and maintaining systolic function and cardiac output. With time, this response becomes maladaptive leading to apoptosis, mediated partly through myocardial ischemia, direct mechanical forces and the actions of angiotensin. Myocardial fibrosis follows the apoptosis, mediated by factors including angiotensin and transforming growth factor- this fibrosis can be seen on a CMR following the administration of gadolinium as "white scar" which is shown here with red arrows. Ultimately this will lead to a dilated and decompensated LV with impaired systolic function. Reproduced with permission from Dweck et al. [2].

Identification of Replacement Fibrosis

CMR is the only non-invasive and radiation-free imaging modality that can be used for myocardial tissue characterization. Using the late gadolinium enhancement (LGE) method and detecting a difference in signal intensity between normal and fibrotic regions, myocardial replacement fibrosis can be correctly identified [16]. Furthermore, in addition to the presence of fibrosis, the location and extent of it can also be demonstrated and quantified with accuracy as shown in Figure 5. In practice, after routine CMR image acquisition of the ventricular myocardium and the valve to allow estimation of the ejection fraction and valve area, patients then receive a standard weight-dependent dose of gadolinium via a peripheral intravenous cannula. Ten to fifteen minutes after the administration, inversion recovery-prepared spoiled gradient echo images are acquired in the standard long and short axis to detect areas of enhancement which appear as "white" [20], as shown in Figures 3 and 5.

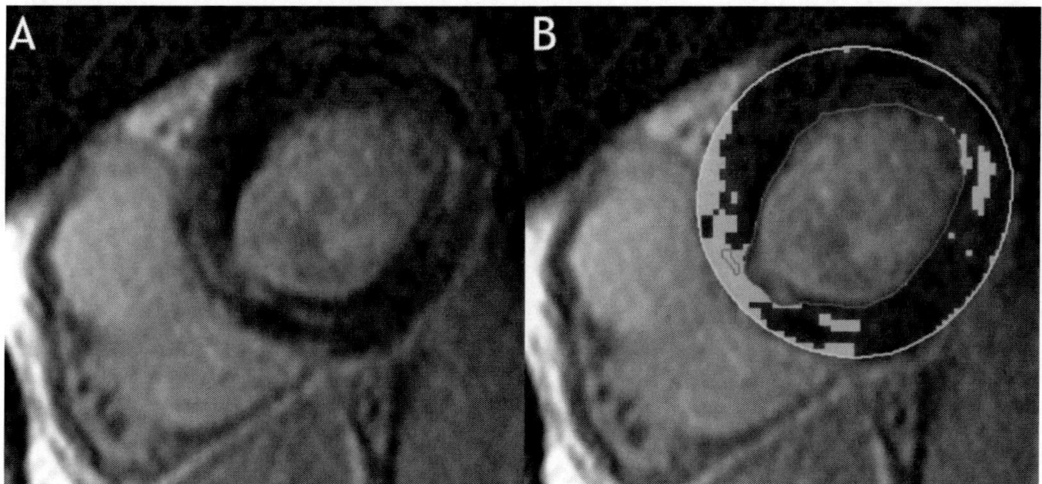

Figure 5. The CMR myocardial image on the left (A) shows myocardial fibrosis which appears as white in a patient with AS. Figure B shows how this fibrosis can be accurately quantified using specific software and expressed as a percentage of the overall LV mass in the same patient. This example was quantified by the Full Width Half Maximum method using CMR42, Circle Cardiovascular Imaging Inc. software and suggested that in this level fibrosis contributed 18% of the myocardial mass.

Significance of Replacement Fibrosis

In the last five years there have been numerous studies supporting the prognostic significance of replacement myocardial fibrosis in patients with AS.

In 2009, Weidemann et al. [19], were the first to report on the importance of myocardial fibrosis in patients with AS. They prospectively investigated 58 patients with severe AS and no coronary disease with echocardiography and CMR (n=46, as 12 patients could not tolerate CMR or it was contraindicated) before and nine months after AVR. Intraoperative myocardial biopsies were also taken for quantification of interstitial fibrosis. Among the patients that could undergo CMR, 18 (39%) showed no fibrosis, 12 (26%) showed mild replacement fibrosis and 16 (35%) showed severe replacement fibrosis; the fibrosis starting usually at the subendocardial layer. At the nine month follow-up, four patients had died (all belonging to the group with severe fibrosis) and ejection fraction was shown to have increased in the subjects with no fibrosis (+8±5%, p=<0.001), remained unchanged in the mild fibrosis group (+2±5%, p=0.42) and showed a trend towards reduction in the severe fibrosis group (-4±2%, p=0.05). The LV mass decreased significantly in all three groups (no fibrosis 24%, mild fibrosis 13%, severe fibrosis 12% all p<0.05), however the absolute decrease was higher in the group with no fibrosis. It was also evident that patients with no fibrosis were more likely to improve symptomatically after AVR than patients with severe fibrosis. Finally, Weidemann et al.'s study also showed that at nine months there was no significant reduction in the degree of replacement fibrosis, suggesting that either the process was irreversible or that it required a longer period for regression.

Azevedo et al. [23] work in 2010 supported Weidemann's findings on the importance of myocardial fibrosis in patients with AS. They prospectively studied a mixed cohort of 54 patients with severe AS and aortic regurgitation with no major epicardial disease, scheduled for AVR with CMR, before and 27 months after AVR. Intraoperative myocardial biopsies were also taken to quantify interstitial fibrosis. A total of 28/54 (52%) required AVR due to AS and 20/28 (72%) showed CMR evidence of delayed enhancement, indicating fibrosis; this correlated well with the histological findings. In this study the improvement in ejection fraction during the follow-up period showed a moderate inverse correlation with the degree of fibrosis (both CMR and histologically). Moreover the authors confirmed that the replacement myocardial fibrosis did not reverse after valve replacement surgery, with repeat CMR scan performed an average of 27 months following surgery. At an extended follow up at 52 months, 16 patients had died. Patients with a larger amount of fibrosis seen both by CMR and histologically demonstrated significantly lower survival probability, further supporting Weidemann's findings.

The prognostic significance of myocardial replacement fibrosis was further confirmed in a study by Dweck et al. [20] in 2011. In this study a mixed population of 143 patients with moderate (40%) or severe (60%) AS with or without coronary disease (45% with coronary disease) referred for CMR in a single institution were prospectively enrolled into a register. Patients were followed up for a mean of two years; during this time 72 patients underwent AVR and 27 died. A total of 49 patients (34%) demonstrated no fibrosis as identified with the late gadolinium enhancement method; 54 (38%) showed midwall fibrosis; and 40 (28%) showed an infarct pattern. Two deaths (both cardiac) occurred in the no fibrosis group; 16 (13 cardiac, out of which three sudden cardiac deaths) died in the midwall fibrosis group; and nine deaths (eight cardiac) were seen in the infarction pattern group, giving a relative percentage of mortality of 4%:30%:23%, respectively. Compared to those with no fibrosis, univariate analysis revealed that patients with midwall fibrosis had an eight-fold increase in all-cause mortality despite similar AS severity and coronary artery disease burden. Patients with an infarct pattern had a six-fold increase. However in a multivariate model, midwall fibrosis (hazard ratio [HR]: 5.35; 95% confidence interval [CI]: 1.16-24.56, p=0.03) and LV ejection fraction (HR: 0.96; 95% CI: 0.94-0.99, p=0.01) were the only independent predictors of all-cause mortality. This was the first study that prospectively identified CMR-determined midwall fibrosis as an independent adverse prognostic factor in patients with AS. Furthermore, this work also supported malignant arrhythmia as a potential explanation of sudden cardiac death in patients with AS, with the midwall fibrosis possibly acting as the source of this arrhythmia [24].

Two papers published in 2012 further supported the prognostic significance of myocardial fibrosis in patients undergoing AVR. Quarto et al. [25] reported on 30-day mortality and major cardiac event (MACE), myocardial infarction and stroke in 63 patients who underwent AVR within 12 months of CMR with gadolinium enhancement. A total of 25 patients (40%) had no fibrosis; 20 (32%) had midwall fibrosis; and 18 (29%) had infarction pattern fibrosis. All the patients without fibrosis were successfully discharged from hospital with no major adverse cardiac events. The midwall fibrosis group had significantly worse peri-operative outcomes compared to both the no fibrosis and infarct groups (p=0.014). Furthermore, at a mean follow-up of two years, five deaths were seen, with three occurring in the midwall fibrosis group and two in the infraction pattern group, confirming that early complications and potentially long-term survival can be affected by the degree of fibrosis. This study was supported by Milano et al. [26] who reported on the long-term survival of 99 patients who underwent AVR and had an intraoperative myocardial biopsy for histological quantification of fibrosis. The patients who survived to be discharged home (n=96) were divided according to the fibrosis burden into absence or mild (n=28), moderate (n=52) and severe (n=19) fibrosis and followed up for a mean of six years (ranging from 1 to 12 years). A total of 32 patients died during this period and the overall actuarial survival at ten years was 53%±6%. Patients with a higher burden of fibrosis demonstrated a significantly lower survival rate at ten years (42%±19% vs. 89%±6%, p=0.002).

Finally, the association of CMR identified myocardial fibrosis and mortality in patients with AS has recently been confirmed by Barone-Rochette et al. [27] In this study 154 patients undergoing surgical AVR were followed up for nearly 3 years. Myocardial fibrosis was demonstrated in 29% of the patients and was associated with worse perioperative mortality and all cause survival with a HR=2.8 on a multivariate model including New York Heart Association (NYHA) classification and left bundle branch block (LBBB).

Interpreted together these studies provide ample evidence that the presence of fibrosis, and particularly midwall pattern, signifies a worse prognosis in patients with moderate or severe AS and that this type of fibrosis is potentially irreversible. However, what remains to be addressed in the next decade is if offering surgery earlier to asymptomatic patients based on the presence and/or burden of replacement fibrosis might improve prognosis. Additionally, patients with AS prior to developing replacement fibrosis have evidence of predominantly interstitial fibrosis. Importantly, and unlike replacement fibrosis, this form of fibrosis might be potentially reversible and cannot usually be identified by the late gadolinium enhancement method as there is no marked demarcation between normal and fibrotic tissue. In the next section, the potential benefit of identifying this earlier form of interstitial fibrosis non-invasively is discussed.

Identification and Significance of Interstitial Fibrosis

Histological studies from intraoperative biopsies at the time of AVR and subsequent follow-up of such patients confirmed that interstitial fibrosis is also associated with a worse prognosis in patients with AS. However, a limiting factor until now has been the difficulty in identifying a suitable, accurate and reproducible method of identifying this type of early fibrosis non-invasively. Messroghli et al. [28] in 2004 first described a novel CMR sequence, the modified Look-Locker inversion recovery (MOLLI), for high-resolution T1 mapping of the heart which made it possible to image interstitial fibrosis as shown in figure 6 panels (B) and (E). Various methods and protocols currently exist for non-invasively measuring interstitial fibrosis which are based on the MOLLI principle. First, native (non-contrast) T1 values can be measured without the need for gadolinium; this is important in various conditions including aortic stenosis, amyloid and myocarditis. Secondly, investigators have measured T1 values after the use of gadolinium, correlating post-contrast T1 with cardiomyopathy, but this can be potentially confounded by the variable renal metabolism of gadolinium in patients. Finally, based on a correction algorithm to incorporate hematocrit, Flett et al. [29] in 2010 firstly reported on the use of both native and post-gadolinium T1 values to calculate the extracellular volume fraction (ECV) percentage which correlated well with histologically quantified interstitial fibrosis from intraoperative biopsies during AVR. Each method has its own advantages as well as limitations, with ECV appearing to have the most potential in assessing interstitial fibrosis in patients with AS [30].

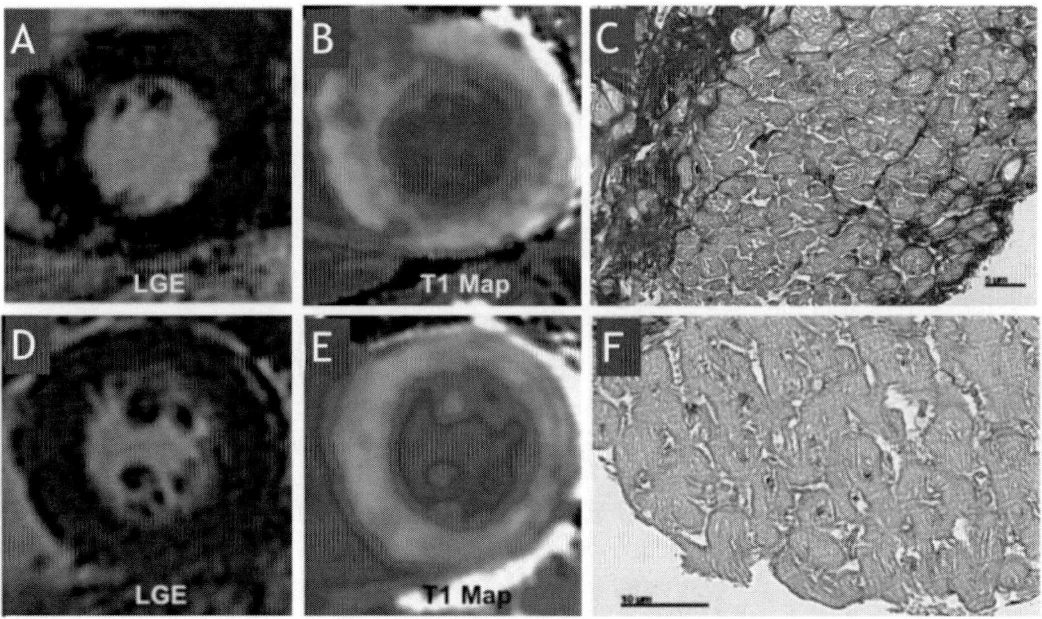

Figure 6. Panel A-C are form one patient with severe AS (peak aortic jet velocity 4.8m/s) and indicate replacement midwall fibrosis (A) and elevated T1 maps (B) on CMR, and extensive collagen staining indicating fibrosis with picrosirius red on myocardial biopsy (C). Despite AS of similar severity (peak aortic jet velocity 5.1m/s), a second patient shown in panels D-F demonstrates normal myocardium with no fibrosis following gadolinium administration (D), lower T1 maps (E) and no histological evidence of fibrosis on myocardial biopsy (F); demonstrating that both replacement and interstitial fibrosis can be accurately assessed non-invasively with CMR and in this case fibrosis is unrelated to the AS severity. Adapted with permission from Chin et al. [31].

Additionally, some early data suggest that ECV can be associated with prognosis in the general population. In particular, Wong et al. [32] performed ECV on a mixed cohort of 793 consecutive patients (range 21.0%-45.8%) and reported on outcomes at ten months. During this time, 39 deaths were noted and 43 patients experienced the composite endpoint of death/ cardiac transplant/ left ventricular assist device implantation. The ECV related to all-cause mortality and the composite endpoint, with every 3% ECV increase conferring a 50%

increase in risk. The same group also reported the following year [33] on patients with type 2 diabetes who had CMR and ECV calculation (n=231) compared with non-diabetic patients (n=945). Patients with diabetes had a higher ECV on average (30.2% vs. 28.1%) and over a median of 1.3 years follow-up, 38 diabetic individuals had events (21 incident hospitalizations for heart failure; 24 deaths), and ECV was associated with these events with a similar 50% increase in risk for every 3% ECV increase.

Unlike the general population or patients with diabetes however, for patients with AS, there have only been small studies to date with limited follow-up data. Flett [34] followed 63 consecutive patients scheduled for surgical AVR with CMR before and six months after AVR. The repeat CMR was only possible in 42 patients. Diffuse (interstitial) myocardial fibrosis was elevated by a factor of 1.5 compared to normal controls. During the follow-up time, six patients died, with five out six having a higher burden of fibrosis. At six months following surgery there was evidence of LV mass regression but a lack of reduction in percentage of diffuse fibrosis.

In summary, myocardial fibrosis is an indicator of LV decompensation in patients with AS, which can potentially predate clinical symptoms or signs. The importance of myocardial replacement fibrosis as an independent prognostic factor in patients with AS, both moderate and severe, has been established. However, further research is required to address whether this should be used as an indicator for earlier AVR in asymptomatic patients. More studies are also needed to conclusively establish the prognostic role of T1/ECV specifically in patients with moderate and severe AS, and whether improvement of ECV can be seen following AVR, as this will be instrumental in determining optimal time for surgery. Furthermore, alongside imaging myocardial fibrosis other established and novel biomarkers could perhaps be successfully used to identify the early transition stages to decompensation in patients with AS.

Markers of LV Decompensation

Symptomatology

According to both European and American guidelines surgery is recommended if a patient has symptoms which are thought to be attributed to the AS (Class I) [21, 22]. Such symptoms typically include angina, syncope or pre-syncope and breathlessness. It is worth remembering however that this triad of symptoms first described by Ross and Braunwald was based on a cohort of relative young patients with predominantly bicuspid and rheumatic AS [8]. With the increasing prevalence of calcific AS in an aging population, milder symptoms in patients with other significant comorbidities might not be adequately appreciated as a sign of early LV decompensation. Therefore, in the asymptomatic patients with severe AS, exercise testing can often be considered.

Exercise Testing

Exercise testing can be undertaken safely in patients with moderate or even severe AS to objectively identify symptoms under standardized conditions. Exercise testing in patients with "asymptomatic" AS can often promptly identify symptoms that are not initially apparent.

Many patients, particularly among the elderly, might unconsciously limit their activities in order to avoid symptoms. Some may also attribute any symptoms they might have to "old age" rather than their AS, and subsequently underreport such symptoms. In a meta-analysis of seven studies involving 491 patients, the sensitivity, specificity, positive and negative predictive values for adverse cardiac events in patients with AS after an abnormal exercise stress test were modest at 75%, 71%, 66% and 79% respectively [35]. Despite this suboptimal sensitivity and specificity both the American [22] and European [21] guidelines recommend that exercise testing could be considered in patients with AS to unmask symptoms which could, in turn, indicate that surgery could be considered (Class I). Intervention can also be considered when a lack of appropriate hemodynamic response to exercise, either a fall in BP (Class IIa) [22] or a failure of BP to increase by >20mmHg (Class IIb) [21].

Echocardiography

Transthoracic echocardiography is the mainstay in the diagnosis and identification of the etiology of AS. It is also very important in identifying both systolic and diastolic function as well as in serial follow up of patients with AS [36]. The EF remains the conventional marker of systolic impairment currently used by both the American and European guidelines. Even in asymptomatic patients, a drop to EF <50% is given a class I of evidence for consideration for surgery in the context of severe AS [21, 22]. One of the limitations of accurate results when using EF in the presence of concentric hypertrophy is the tendency for this to be overestimated- due to increase in myocardial wall thickness and filling pressures alongside a reduction in ventricular volumes- resulting in normal or even supernormal EF despite significant impairment in intrinsic myocardial contractility [37, 38]. In addition, echocardiography can be used to assess diastolic function [39]. Traditionally this was done using the Doppler mitral inflow and myocardial tissue velocities but it did not have an impact on determining the timing of surgery.

With more advanced echocardiographic techniques including strain and strain rate using 2D speckle tracking, it is possible that this will lead to earlier detection of LV dysfunction, and subsequently, earlier consideration for surgery. Serial echocardiography can also assess the rate of progression of stenosis, with an annual rate of progression of >0.3m/s/year attracting a class IIa indication for surgery in the European guidelines [21]. This is also supported in the American guidelines where for low risk patients with rapid progression of AS but who remain asymptomatic a class IIb indication for surgery has been given [22]. Patients who remain asymptomatic but with very severe AS defined as peak transvalvular gradient of 5.5m/s (peak gradient 120mmHg) have a IIa indication for surgery as well [21]. Therefore, although echocardiography plays a crucial role in the diagnosis of AS, its role in identifying the appropriate timing for surgery remains limited- it is mainly used for identifying patients whose EF has already deteriorated, dropping to <50% which is a late stage of LV decompensation. Complementing echocardiography, peripheral blood biomarkers might also be utilized in an attempt to better identify an earlier stage of LV decompensation and prior to the transition from hypertrophy to heart failure which could aid in identifying the optimal timing for surgery and are discussed in the following section.

Blood Biomarkers of Ventricular Decompensation in Aortic Stenosis

There is growing interest in the use of blood biomarkers for assessing disease severity and prognosis in AS and in particular in identifying the transition to hypertrophy and failure.

Brain Natriuretic Peptide and N-Terminal-proBNP

Brain natriuretic peptide and NT-proBNP are endogenous cardiac hormones (made up of 32-amino acids and 76-amino acid, respectively) that are released in response to LV wall stress and decompensated LV function. Elevated levels of BNP and NT-proBNP have been demonstrated in patients with symptomatic AS [40, 41]. There is much debate about the role of these biomarkers in providing sound prognostic information however, particularly as they are known to increase with aging and therefore the normal range can be difficult to define. In severe AS, NT-proBNP has been shown to supplement clinical and echocardiographic findings, providing useful prognostic information such as symptom-free survival and postoperative survival rates and LV function.

The other main question surrounding the use of BNP and NT-proBNP is whether they could play a role in assessing the severity and prognosis in patients with asymptomatic AS. BNP levels have been reported as an independent predictor of outcome (along with female sex and peak aortic-jet velocity) in patients with asymptomatic AS, thus helping identify which patients will benefit from early surgical intervention [42, 43]. However, further work has disputed this by demonstrating that outcomes are not significantly worse with elevated NT-proBNP levels when the analysis is adjusted for age, gender and severity of AS; making the routine use of BNP and NT-proBNP currently to guide the time for surgery less clear.

High-Sensitivity Troponin

Cardiac troponin is a structural protein present in the myocardium. Elevated concentrations of plasma troponin are a specific indicator of myocardial injury independently of etiology.

Recent advances in assay technology have improved the sensitivity of plasma troponin testing and detectable lower plasma troponin concentrations have opened the door for its use in AS. Although BNP can identify myocardial dysfunction, high-sensitivity troponin is associated with increased myocardial injury and LV decompensation.

Through CMR it has recently been shown that patients with increased high-sensitivity troponin I have evidence of LV decompensation with increased LV mass and myocardial fibrosis, independently of coronary artery disease. Moreover in an asymptomatic population with AS, high-sensitivity troponin has recently been associated with a higher chance of requiring AVR and cardiovascular mortality [31].

Troponins could therefore play an important role in the identification of potentially early LV dysfunction and thus further guide towards the optimal time for surgery- however, while early studies show promising results, further research is required to identify the exact role that troponins could play in routine clinical care.

Other Novel Blood Biomarkers

Finally two more promising biomarkers have recently been studied in patients with AS. Galectin-3, a member of the lectin family, is a novel biomarker which has shown potential to provide prognostic information in patients with acute decompensated and chronic heart failure [44]. Fibroblast and macrophage activation, a characteristic feature of fibrosis and cardiac remodeling, occurs in response to galectin-3 upregulation in heart failure. Myocardial fibrosis and remodeling are thought to be important prognostic features in AS, therefore galectin-3 could hold potential as a useful prognostic marker in AS. Another novel biomarker of myocardial fibrosis with potential as a marker of severity and prognosis in AS is ST2 [45]. It is a member of the interleukin-1 receptor family and has been implicated in the process of cardiac fibrosis and ventricular dysfunction.

Although both ST2 and Galectin-3 show positive signs of becoming new biomarkers that can be useful in identifying early signs of LV decompensation, there is still a long way to go before they can be used routinely in clinical practice.

Clinical Vignettes of Patients with AS, Hypertrophy and Fibrosis

It is not always an easy task to identify the optimal timing for recommending surgery in patients with AS. Too early and patients are unnecessarily exposed to the risk of surgery and either anticoagulation or bioprosthetic valve degeneration. Too late and irreversible myocardial damage occurs with long term prognostic implications. Through the following vignettes we will discuss the therapeutic options for patients with AS particularly in the context of hypertrophy and fibrosis.

Case 1: A 65 year old woman with known asymptomatic severe AS is reviewed routinely in the cardiology outpatient clinic. She claims to exercise frequently including cycling 2-3 km daily with no symptoms. Her echocardiographic parameters have worsened only marginally in the last 6 months with peak gradient 75mmHg, mean gradient 42mmHg, AVA 0.9mm and EF=58%. She is feeling very well and currently has an excellent quality of life. She likes to read articles relating to AS both on the internet and freely available medical journals. Although she is not keen for surgery at present she is worried that the optimal window for surgery might be missed. She asks if there are any further tests that should/ could be done to confirm that there is no current need for surgery.

The timing for surgical intervention for patients with AS is crucial. On the one hand operating early reduces the risks associated with surgery. On the other hand however, this forces patients to live with a prosthetic valve and its comorbidities for longer. More worryingly, delaying surgery until the LV has decompensated means that the patient is both at higher risk during surgery but also might not derive good symptomatic improvement (if they had symptoms) following surgery.

This patient does not fulfill any of the current guidelines for consideration of surgery. Although she does have echocardiographic parameters of severe AS, she remains asymptomatic and, as such, not a candidate for surgery at present. However, recent research has suggested that earlier surgery in asymptomatic patients might lead to reduced overall cardiac mortality in the longer term [46], although this practice is not reflected in the current guidelines [21, 22].

It could be beneficial to undertake formal exercise testing or even exercise echocardiography to formally assess symptoms and exercise capacity as well as changes in the LV function with exercise. Despite the claim of regular exercise, it is possible that she may not be achieving a high enough cardiovascular effect to prompt symptoms (e.g., cycling on flat surface at a very low speed-low impact exercise). To ensure that the patient is truly asymptomatic she could undergo a supervised exercise test to confirm the lack of symptoms but also be monitored for appropriate blood pressure response. If either of these is shown to be unsatisfactory (symptoms developing or poor exercise capacity) or there is inappropriate response of BP (decrease in BP according to European guidance [21], lack of increase by >20mmHg according to American guidance [22]) then surgery could be considered.

Furthermore, BNP and highly sensitive troponin could be measured in the blood- if both are within normal limits this will be extremely reassuring. If either is elevated however, this could raise concern that the timing for surgery is approaching and prompt closer follow up, i.e., seeing the patient in outpatients in a 2-3 months with repeat rest transthoracic echocardiogram and blood tests.

A CMR should also be considered. If this shows normal myocardial characterization with no myocardial replacement fibrosis following gadolinium administration, then this will be reassuring. If however there is abnormal enhancement suggestive of fibrosis it could alert clinicians that the timing for surgery is nearing and result in more frequent reviews of the patient in clinic.

Case 2: A 75 year old man, with well controlled hypertension is known to have moderate to severe trileaflet calcific AS for the last three years. His echocardiogram shows normal systolic function (EF=65%), mild hypertrophy, with a mean gradient of 44mmHg and peak gradient of 72mmHg. For the last three months he is getting some breathlessness when walking briskly, for example when trying to catch a bus.

In this scenario we have a patient with previously known moderate/ severe aortic stenosis which has progressed and it is now in the severe range. His systolic function is also normal and the absence of significant comorbidities puts him in a low risk for cardiac surgery with a EUROSCORE II calculated at 0.85% (the EUROSCORE is a validated method of predicting the chance of dying during or shortly after undergoing heart surgery and it is reported as an absolute percentage value). Following clinical examination, if the symptoms of breathlessness are thought to relate to the AS (i.e., other conditions have been excluded such as chronic obstructive pulmonary disease, pneumonia, anemia, etc.) then he should be considered for elective aortic valve replacement (Class I). It is known that significant delay will lead to decompensation of his LV function and adversely affect his long-term prognosis but also the success of symptomatic improvement after surgery, therefore an early elective surgical slot would be desirable.

Case 3: A 47 year old woman with known asymptomatic severe bicuspid AS is reviewed routinely in the outpatient clinic. She remains asymptomatic and she has no other medical conditions. Her last echocardiogram six months previously had shown a peak gradient of 82mmHg, mean gradient 41mmHg and AVA 0.9 cm^2 and EF 55%. Her echocardiogram today has shown peak gradient 75mmHg, mean gradient 38mmHg and AVA 0.8cm^2. Her EF has dropped to 42%.

Here we have a patient who is being reviewed in the cardiology outpatient clinic regularly, who has no significant comorbidities and remains asymptomatic. Her EF has however decreased significantly. If this is thought to relate to AS it would suggest that LV has begun to decompensate relatively rapidly. Despite this she still remains a very good surgical candidate with EUROSCORE II calculated at 0.85 %. Unless surgery is undertaken (Class I) significant deterioration in EF is likely to follow making subsequent valve surgery more risky. Assuming that surgery is delayed for a few months and her EF drops further to <30% then her EUROSCORE II will increase to 1.38% (a relative increase of 62%) indicating the importance of the optimal window for undertaking surgery. It would also be important to image the aorta looking for aortopathy that potentially complicates a bicuspid aortic valve, as this could be corrected at the time of surgery.

Case 4: A 62 year old man with known asymptomatic severe AS is reviewed routinely in clinic. His echocardiogram shows peak gradient 93mmHg, mean gradient 50mmHg and AVA 0.7cm^2, EF 72% and septal wall thickness is 17mm. He undergoes CMR which confirms the hypertrophy and elevated mass. His family doctor has enquired whether surgery should be offered.

Given his asymptomatic status there is no urgency in considering AV surgery. However, a IIb indication exists for surgery in patients with asymptomatic AS and severe LVH [22]. Therefore, surgery could be justified according to the guidance. It would be important to further risk stratify this patient with an exercise test ideally with echocardiography before and after the exercise, and blood tests including BNP and high-sensitivity troponin. If either of these is abnormal it could suggest that the patient is at risk of decompensating and therefore surgery could be considered. Although the guidance would support a class IIb for intervening many clinicians might still consider that this is not yet the time for surgery and often look for other signs of decompensation at this stage to further support a decision prior to referral for surgery.

Case 5: An 82 year old woman with significant comorbidities has been admitted as an emergency with symptoms and signs of heart failure. She had a coronary artery bypass graft six years previously receiving a LIMA (left internal mammary artery) graft to the LAD (left anterior descending artery) and two vein grafts to the circumflex and right coronary artery. Other comorbidities include moderate renal impairment, insulin treated diabetes, high BMI=37, 50 pack-year smoking history and poor mobility using a wheelchair following a road traffic accident. On cardiac auscultation an ejection systolic murmur over the aortic area with absent second heart sound was identified. A transthoracic echocardiogram showed a trileaflet valve which was severely stenosed with peak gradient 122mmHg, mean gradient 60mmHg and AVA=0.4cm^2. Her EF was 48% and there was significant LVH. Both the patient and the family are adamant that she has very good quality of life and keen to explore any therapeutic options.

This patient represents a complex case. With an aging population it is anticipated that the prevalence of patients with AS and significant comorbidities will increase. Without any intervention on the aortic valve her life expectancy is a few months and likely during this period she will have multiple hospital admissions. Apart from heart failure medication that could control some of the symptoms there is no medical therapy that will improve prognosis. Intervention to the aortic valve is warranted and this could take the form of aortic valve valvuloplasty, TAVI (transcatheter aortic valve implantation) or surgical valve replacement. There is significant evidence that balloon valvuloplasty will not prolong her life but might improve her quality of life with reduced hospitalizations. Surgery on the other hand will not be without risk. In view of her comorbidities the EUROSCORE II is very high at 25%. This would represent significant risk and also an open procedure could also damage the LIMA graft. The attractive option for this patient would be a TAVI. This could be achieved either completely percutaneously or even transapically at reduced risk compared to the surgical option. Furthermore, this could be undertaken as a staged procedure offering the patient balloon valvuloplasty initially so the patient can improve from her heart failure and then come back for completion and valve implantation. Given her high EUROSCORE, it would seem very appropriate to discuss this case in a Heart Team meeting, and if valve anatomy is suitable for a percutaneous option then TAVI could be offered (indication I).

Conclusion

In summary, patients with AS develop a LV hypertrophic response that is initially adaptive. However with time this process decompensates due to progressive myocyte cell death and myocardial fibrosis and patients transition to symptoms, heart failure and adverse cardiovascular events. It is imperative to look for early evidence of decompensation and identify the optimal window for surgical intervention for each patient; this will minimize the operative risk whilst allowing the patients to have better cardiac remodeling following surgery. Currently history and clinical examination represent the cornerstone of this approach, with the identification of symptoms related to AS such as breathlessness, chest pain, syncope and pre-syncope the key to identifying LV decompensation. Unfortunately in the elderly the assessment of symptoms is frequently challenging and where appropriate assessment of LV systolic function, and exercise tolerance testing in particular should also be considered. None of these approaches are however perfect and there is considerable interest in the development of novel more objective biomarkers of LV decompensation, including CMR and blood biomarkers such as troponin and BNP that may improve this decision-making process.

References

[1]   Lindroos M, Kupari M, Heikkilä J, Tilvis R. Prevalence of aortic valve abnormalities in the elderly: an echocardiographic study of a random population sample. *J. Am. Coll. Cardiol.* 1993;21(5):1220-5. Available at: http://www.ncbi.nlm.nih.gov/pubmed/8459080.

[2]   Dweck MR, Boon N a, Newby DE. Calcific aortic stenosis: a disease of the valve and the myocardium. *J. Am. Coll. Cardiol.* 2012;60(19):1854-63. doi:10.1016/j.jacc.2012.02.093.

[3]   Dunning J, Gao H, Chambers J, et al. Aortic valve surgery: marked increases in volume and significant decreases in mechanical valve use--an analysis of 41,227 patients over 5 years from the Society for Cardiothoracic Surgery in Great Britain and Ireland National database. *J. Thorac. Cardiovasc. Surg.* 2011;142(4):776-782.e3. doi:10.1016/j.jtcvs.2011.04.048.

[4]   Carabello B. The relationship of left ventricular geometry and hypertrophy to left ventricular function in valvular heart disease. *J. Hear. Valve. Dis.* 1995;S2:S132-8.

[5]   Yarbrough W, Mukherjee R, Ikonomidis J, Zile M, Spinale F. NIH Public Access. *J. Thorac. Cardiovasc. Surg.* 2012;143(3):656-664.doi:10.1016/j.jtcvs.2011.04.044. Myocardial.

[6]   Gunther S, Grossman W. Determinants of ventricular function in pressure-overload hypertrophy in man. *Circulation.* 1979;59(4):679-688. doi:10.1161/01.CIR.59.4.679.

[7]   Kupari M, Turto H, Lommi J. Left ventricular hypertrophy in aortic valve stenosis: preventive or promotive of systolic dysfunction and heart failure? *Eur. Heart J.* 2005;26(17):1790-6. doi:10.1093/eurheartj/ehi290.

[8]   Chin CW, Vassiliou V, Jenkins WS, Prasad SK, Newby DE, Dweck MR. Markers of left ventricular decompensation in aortic stenosis. *Expert Rev. Cardiovasc. Ther.* 2014;12(7):901-12. doi:10.1586/14779072.2014.923307.

[9]   Dweck MR, Joshi S, Murigu T, et al. Left ventricular remodeling and hypertrophy in patients with aortic stenosis: insights from cardiovascular magnetic resonance. *J. Cardiovasc. Magn. Reson.* 2012;14(1):50. doi:10.1186/1532-429X-14-50.

[10] Seiler C, Jenni R. Severe aortic stenosis without left ventricular hypertrophy: prevalence, predictors, and short-term follow up after aortic valve replacement. *Heart.* 1996;76(3):250-5. Available at: http://www.pubmedcentral.nih.gov/articlerender.fcgi? artid=484516&tool=pmcentrez&rendertype=abstract.

[11] Carroll JD, Carroll EP, Feldman T, et al. Sex-associated differences in left ventricular function in aortic stenosis of the elderly. *Circulation.* 1992;86(4):1099-1107. doi:10.1161/01.CIR.86.4.1099.

[12] Regitz-Zagrosek V, Oertelt-Prigione S, Seeland U, Hetzer R. Sex and Gender Differences in Myocardial Hypertrophy and Heart Failure. *Circ. J.* 2010;74(7):1265-1273. doi:10.1253/circj.CJ-10-0196.

[13] Montgomery H. Editorial Should the contribution of ACE gene polymorphism to left ventricular hypertrophy be reconsidered ? *Heart.* 1997;6:489-490.

[14] Beach JM, Mihaljevic T, Rajeswaran J, et al. Ventricular hypertrophy and left atrial dilatation persist and are associated with reduced survival after valve replacement for aortic stenosis. *J. Thorac. Cardiovasc. Surg.* 2014;147(1):362-369.e8. doi:10.1016/j.jtcvs.2012.12.016.

[15] Levy D, Garriso RJ, Savvage DD, Kannel WB, Catselli WP. Prognostic Implications of echocardiographically determined left ventricular mass in the framingham study. *New Englanf. J. Med.* 1990;322(22):1561-66.

[16] McCrohon J a, Moon JCC, Prasad SK, et al. Differentiation of heart failure related to dilated cardiomyopathy and coronary artery disease using gadolinium-enhanced cardiovascular magnetic resonance. *Circulation.* 2003;108(1):54-9. doi:10.1161/01.CIR.0000078641.19365.4C.

[17] Mahrholdt H, Wagner A, Judd RM, Sechtem U, Kim RJ. Delayed enhancement cardiovascular magnetic resonance assessment of non-ischaemic cardiomyopathies. *Eur Heart J.* 2005;26(15):1461-74. doi:10.1093/eurheartj/ehi258.

[18] Hein S, Arnon E, Kostin S, et al. Progression From Compensated Hypertrophy to Failure in the Pressure-Overloaded Human Heart: Structural Deterioration and Compensatory Mechanisms. *Circulation.* 2003;107(7):984-991. doi:10.1161 /01.CIR. 0000051865.66123.B7.

[19] Weidemann F, Herrmann S, Störk S, et al. Impact of myocardial fibrosis in patients with symptomatic severe aortic stenosis. *Circulation*. 2009;120(7):577-84. doi:10.1161/CIRCULATIONAHA.108.847772.

[20] Dweck MR, Joshi S, Murigu T, et al. Midwall fibrosis is an independent predictor of mortality in patients with aortic stenosis. *J. Am. Coll. Cardiol*. 2011;58(12):1271-9. doi:10.1016/j.jacc.2011.03.064.

[21] Vahanian A, Alfieri O, Andreotti F, et al. Guidelines on the management of valvular heart disease (version 2012). *Eur. Heart J*. 2012;33(19):2451-96. doi:10.1093/eurheartj/ehs109.

[22] Nishimura R a, Otto CM, Bonow RO, et al. 2014 AHA/ACC Guideline for the Management of Patients With Valvular Heart Disease: Executive Summary: A Report of the American College of Cardiology/American Heart Association Task Force on Practice Guidelines. *J. Am. Coll. Cardiol*. 2014;online fir. doi:10.1016/ j.jacc.2014.02.537.

[23] Azevedo CF, Nigri M, Higuchi ML, et al. Prognostic significance of myocardial fibrosis quantification by histopathology and magnetic resonance imaging in patients with severe aortic valve disease. *J. Am. Coll. Cardiol*. 2010;56(4):278-87. doi:10.1016/j.jacc.2009.12.074.

[24] Nazarian S. Is ventricular arrhythmia a possible mediator of the association between aortic stenosis-related midwall fibrosis and mortality? *J. Am. Coll. Cardiol*. 2011;58(12):1280-2. doi:10.1016/j.jacc.2011.04.045.

[25] Quarto C, Dweck MR, Murigu T, et al. Late gadolinium enhancement as a potential marker of increased perioperative risk in aortic valve replacement. *Interact Cardiovasc Thorac. Surg*. 2012;15(1):45-50. doi:10.1093/icvts/ivs098.

[26] Milano AD, Faggian G, Dodonov M, et al. Prognostic value of myocardial fibrosis in patients with severe aortic valve stenosis. *J. Thorac. Cardiovasc. Surg*. 2012;144(4):830-7. doi:10.1016/j.jtcvs.2011.11.024.

[27] Barone-Rochette G, Piérard S, De Meester de Ravenstein C, et al. Prognostic Significance of LGE by CMR in Aortic Stenosis Patients Undergoing Valve Replacement. *J. Am. Coll. Cardiol*. 2014;64(2):144-154. doi:10.1016/ j.jacc.2014.02.612.

[28] Messroghli DR, Radjenovic A, Kozerke S, Higgins DM, Sivananthan MU, Ridgway JP. Modified Look-Locker inversion recovery (MOLLI) for high-resolution T1 mapping of the heart. *Magn. Reson. Med*. 2004;52(1):141-6. doi:10.1002/mrm.20110.

[29] Flett AS, Hayward MP, Ashworth MT, et al. Equilibrium contrast cardiovascular magnetic resonance for the measurement of diffuse myocardial fibrosis: preliminary validation in humans. *Circulation*. 2010;122(2):138-44. doi:10.1161/ CIRCULATIONAHA.109.930636.

[30] Chin CW, Semple S, Malley T, et al. Optimization and comparison of myocardial T1 techniques at 3T in patients with aortic stenosis. *Eur. Heart J. Cardiovasc Imaging*. 2014:15(5):555-556. doi:10.1093/ehjci/jet245.

[31] Chin CW, Shah AS V, McAllister D a, et al. High-sensitivity troponin I concentrations are a marker of an advanced hypertrophic response and adverse outcomes in patients with aortic stenosis. *Eur. Heart J*. 2014;35(34):2312-2321. doi:10.1093/eurheartj/ ehu189.

[32] Wong TC, Piehler K, Meier CG, et al. Association between extracellular matrix expansion quantified by cardiovascular magnetic resonance and short-term mortality. *Circulation.* 2012;126(10):1206-16. doi:10.1161/CIRCULATIONAHA.111.089409.

[33] Wong TC, Piehler KM, Kang I a, et al. Myocardial extracellular volume fraction quantified by cardiovascular magnetic resonance is increased in diabetes and associated with mortality and incident heart failure admission. *Eur. Heart J.* 2013;3(Mi):1-8. doi:10.1093/eurheartj/eht193.

[34] Flett AS, Sado DM, Quarta G, et al. Diffuse myocardial fibrosis in severe aortic stenosis: an equilibrium contrast cardiovascular magnetic resonance study. *Eur. Heart J. Cardiovasc. Imaging.* 2012;13(10):819-26. doi:10.1093/ehjci/jes102.

[35] Rafique AM, Biner S, Ray I, Forrester JS, Tolstrup K, Siegel RJ. Meta-Analysis of Prognostic Value of Stress Testing in Patients With Asymptomatic Severe Aortic Stenosis. *AJC.* 2009;104(7):972-977. doi:10.1016/j.amjcard.2009.05.044.

[36] Lancellotti P, Donal E, Magne J, et al. Impact of global left ventricular afterload on left ventricular function in asymptomatic severe aortic stenosis: a two-dimensional speckle-tracking study. *Eur. J. Echocardiogr.* 2010;11(6):537-43. doi:10.1093 /ejechocard/jeq014.

[37] Pibarot P, Dumesnil JG. Improving assessment of aortic stenosis. *J Am Coll Cardiol.* 2012;60(3):169-80. doi:10.1016/j.jacc.2011.11.078.

[38] Dumesnil JG, Shoucri RM. Effect of the geometry of the left ventricle on the calculation of ejection fraction. *Circulation.* 1982;65(1):91-98. doi:10.1161/ 01.CIR.65.1.91.

[39] Bruch C, Stypmann J, Grude M, Gradaus R, Breithardt G, Wichter T. Tissue Doppler imaging in patients with moderate to severe aortic valve stenosis: clinical usefulness and diagnostic accuracy. *Am. Heart J.* 2004;148(4):696-702. doi:10.1016/ j.ahj.2004.03.049.

[40] Weber M, Arnold R, Rau M, et al. Relation of N-terminal pro-B-type natriuretic peptide to severity of valvular aortic stenosis. *Am. J. Cardiol.* 2004;94(6):740-5. doi:10.1016/j.amjcard.2004.05.055.

[41] Ben-Dor I, Minha S, Barbash IM, et al. Correlation of brain natriuretic peptide levels in patients with severe aortic stenosis undergoing operative valve replacement or percutaneous transcatheter intervention with clinical, echocardiographic, and hemodynamic factors and prognosis. *Am. J. Cardiol.* 2013;112(4):574-9. doi:10.1016/j.amjcard.2013.04.023.

[42] Monin J-L, Lancellotti P, Monchi M, et al. Risk score for predicting outcome in patients with asymptomatic aortic stenosis. *Circulation.* 2009;120(1):69-75. doi:10.1161/CIRCULATIONAHA.108.808857.

[43] Cimadevilla C, Cueff C, Hekimian G, et al. Prognostic value of B-type natriuretic peptide in elderly patients with aortic valve stenosis: the COFRASA-GENERAC study. *Heart.* 2013;99(7):461-7. doi:10.1136/heartjnl-2012-303284.

[44] Sharma UC, Pokharel S, van Brakel TJ, et al. Galectin-3 marks activated macrophages in failure-prone hypertrophied hearts and contributes to cardiac dysfunction. *Circulation.* 2004;110(19):3121-8. doi:10.1161/01.CIR.0000147181.65298.4D.

[45] Breyley JG, Novak E, Wittenberg AM, et al. Soluble St2 Is Associated With Increased Mortality and Reclassifies Risk in Patients With Severe Aortic Stenosis. *J. Am. Coll. Cardiol.* 2014;63(12):A1920. doi:10.1016/S0735-1097(14)61923-9.

[46] Kang D-H, Park S-J, Rim JH, et al. Early surgery versus conventional treatment in asymptomatic very severe aortic stenosis. *Circulation.* 2010;121(13):1502-9. doi:10.1161/CIRCULATIONAHA.109.909903.

ISBN: 978-1-63463-022-1
© 2015 Nova Science Publishers, Inc.

Chapter 3

Left Ventricular Hypertrophy in Chronic Kidney Disease Patients

Luca Di Lullo, M.D., Ph.D.
Department of Nephrology and Dialysis – "L. Parodi Delfino Hospital" –
Colleferro, Rome, Italy

Abstract

Cardiovascular diseases such as coronary artery disease, congestive heart failure, arrhtyhmias and sudden cardiac death represent main causes of morbidity and mortality in patients with chronic kidney disease (CKD). Pathogenesis includes close linkage between heart and kidneys and involves traditional and non-traditional risk factors. According to well – established classification of cardio – renal syndrome, cardiovascular involvement in chronic kidney disease is known as "Type 4 Cardio – Renal Syndrome" (chronic reno – cardiac).

Uremic cardiopathy is mainly characterized by both left ventricular systolic and diastolic impairment, often associated to right heart dysfunction due to presence of vascular access for hemodialysis.

Typical clinical picture is represented by left ventricular hypertrophy (LVH), which pathogenesis is multifactorial and closely linked to elevated blood pressure, vascular stiffness and atherosclerosis.

Diagnosis is mainly provided by ultrasound (2D and 3D echocardiography) and cardiac magnetic resonance imaging (CMRI), although echocardiography is most widely employed because it's non – invasive and cheaper than CMRI.

The following chapter makes an overview about epidemiology, pathophysiology, diagnosis and treatment key features of left ventricular hypertrophy CKD patients

1. Introduction

Cardiovascular diseases such as coronary artery disease, congestive heart failure, arrhtyhmias and sudden cardiac death represent main causes of morbidity and mortality in patients with chronic kidney disease (CKD). According to well – established classification of cardio – renal syndrome, cardiovascular involvement in chronic kidney disease is known as "Type 4 Cardio – Renal Syndrome" (chronic reno – cardiac).

Term known as "Cardio Renal Syndrome" (CRS) includes broad spectrum of diseases in which heart and kidney are both involved. Consensus conference of Acute Dialysis Quality Initiative Group [1] recently proposed term "cardio - renal syndrome" (CRS) to define clinical overlap between kidney and heart dysfunction. A clear classification of CRS is crucial as its wide, correct application is required to allow correct interactions between cardiologists and nephrologists.

CRS classification (figure 1) essentially recognizes two main groups, cardio - renal and reno - cardiac CRS, on the basis of primum movens of disease (cardiac or renal), then divided into acute and chronic according to disease's onset.

Left ventricular hypertrophy represent key feature in uremic cardiopathy and it's related to type – 4 CRS, chronic reno – cardiac cardiorenal syndrome.

Cardiovascular complications can occur at any stage of chronic kidney disease (CKD) independently by GFR (glomerular filtration rate) levels.

Type – 4 CRS definition itself involves that is required kidney disease before development of heart failure and this is not always possible.

Cardiorenal syndrome classification

Cardiorenal Syndrome (CRS) General Definition:
A pathophysiologic disorder of the heart and kidneys whereby acute or chronic dysfunction in one organ may induce acute or chronic dysfunction in the other organ
CRS Type I (Acute Cardiorenal Syndrome)
Abrupt worsening of cardiac function (e.g. acute cardiogenic shock or acutely decompensated congestive heart failure) leading to acute kidney injury
CRS Type II (Chronic Cardiorenal Syndrome)
Chronic abnormalities in cardiac function (e.g. chronic congestive heart failure) causing progressive and potentially permanent chronic kidney disease
CRS Type III (Acute Renocardiac Syndrome)
Abrupt worsening of renal function (e.g. acute kidney ischaemia or glomerulonephritis) causing acute cardiac disorder (e.g. heart failure, arrhythmia, ischemia)
CRS Type IV (Chronic Renocardiac Syndrome)
Chronic kidney disease (e.g. chronic glomerular or interstitial disease) contributing to decreased cardiac function, cardiac hypertrophy and/or increased risk of adverse cardiovascular events
CRS Type V (Secondary Cardiorenal Syndrome)
Systemic condition (e.g. diabetes mellitus, sepsis) causing both cardiac and renal dysfunction

Figure 1. Classification of cardiorenal syndrome.

2. Epidemiology

It's now clear close relationship between CKD and increased risk for cardiovascular disease; major cardiac events actually representing almost 50 % death causes in CKD patients [2].

Since early stages of CKD to end stage renal disease (ESRD) cardiovascular involvement is present, in part due to aging population, in part linked to higher rates of diabetic, dyslipidemic and hypertensive patients among CKD population [3].

The HEMO Study clearly demonstrated high prevalence (about 80%) of cardiovascular disease in hemodialysis patients in relation with age, prevalence of diabetes and dialysis duration [4]: most of patients were hospitalized for acute coronary syndrome.

Stage I – IV CKD patients show lower degrees of cardiovascular involvement in respect of dialysis (both hemodialysis and peritoneal dialysis) ones with dose – related relationship becoming more evident as GFR falls below 60 ml/min/1.73 m^2 [5, 6].

Meta – analysis by Tonelli et al., [7] conducted on 1.4 million patients found higher mortality rates for all causes with eGFR decline with relative death odds ratio of 1.9, 2.6 and 4.4 for GFR levels of 80, 60 and 40 ml/min, respectively.

Cardiovascular risk is particularly evident in patients with stage IIIb – IV (according to K/DOQI CKD classifcation) renal disease and in those underwent renal replacement therapy (hemodialysis, peritoneal dialysis and transplant) [8]

Risk of adverse cardiovascular events, compared to control group with normal GFR, was 43 percent higher in patients with GFR between 45 – 59 ml/min/1.73 m^2 and 343 percent higher in those with GFR under 15 ml/min/1.73 m^2. Stage V CKD patients, not on renal replacement therapy, showed mortality rates similar to those on dialysis therapy [9]. It's actually possible to estimate that cardiovascular diseases account for 50 % deaths in CKD patients regardless of biological age [10].

Kidney Early Evaluation Program (KEEP) enrolled and screened about 100,000 people for kidney disease reporting various comorbid disease including congestive heart failure; analysis showed risk for cardiovascular disease incresing by 15 percent for every increasing stage of CKD [11].

Chronic Renal Insufficiency Cohort (CRIC) Study investigators focused their attention on 190 patients presenting stage III to end - stage renal disease and performing serial echocardiographic exams; in two - years evaluation period in which patients shifted from stage V to end – stage renal disease, ejection fraction (EF) dropped from 53 to 50 percent; therefore they found that subjects with EF less than 50 percent increased by 20 percent [12].

Cardiovascular events are not only restricted to end – stage renal disease, but early CKD stages are also associated with variable degrees of heart failure as underlined in the ARIC (Atherosclerosis Risk in Communities) population study [13] focused on incident cardiovascular events (subjects with pre – existing heart failure were dropped out) in about 15,000 subjects. Statistical analysis found an increase in heart failure in subjects with eGFR less than 60 ml/min/1.73 m^2.

Cox analysis demonstrated relative hazard of incident heart failure by 1.10 in subjects with GFR range of 60 – 89 ml/min/1.73 m^2 and 1.94 in those with GFR lower than 60 ml/min/1.73 m^2.

Prevalence of LVH varies from 16 to 31% in individuals with GFR >30 ml/min, increasing to 60–75% prior to starting renal replacement therapy, and up to 90% of patients after the initiation of dialysis [14]. Foley et al. [15] noted that 74% of patients had echocardiographic evidence of LVH with over 30% having concurrent LV failure and Foley himself [16] followed 596 incident hemodialysis patients with no prior history of cardiac disease to investigate whether incidence of LVH correlates with duration of dialysis and demonstrated, after 18 months of dialysis, a 62% increase of LMVI with 49% patients developing overt LV failure. These observations raise the question of whether the very process of dialysis facilitates the development of LVH in ESRD patients.

3. Pathophysiology of Left Ventricular Hyperthrophy in Chronic Kidney Disease

Echocardiographic abnormalities (impairment of ejection fraction, increased end – systolic and end – disatolic left ventricular diameter and volume) are frequently reported since early stages of CKD to end – stage renal disease.

The pathogenetic factors involved in LV hypertrophy CKD and ESRD have generally been divided into three categories [17 – 19]: (1) afterload related, (2) preload related and (3) not afterload or preload related. First ones are represented by increase in systemic arterial resistance, elevated arterial blood pressure, and reduced large-vessel compliance [17 – 20] related in part to aortic "calcification" typical in CKD patients; all these factors result in myocardial cell thickening and concentric LV remodeling often together with activation of the intracardiac renin-angiotensin system [19, 21]. Oxidative stress and xanthine oxidase activation may be also involved in LVH [22] such as phosphodiesterase-5 pathway as demonstrated by pharmacological effects of sildenafil therapy that attenuates LVH [23]. Among preload-related factors we have to underline the role of intravascular volume expansion (salt and fluid loading), secondary anemia and presence arterio-venous fistulas [14, 24, 25], resulting in myocardial cell lengthening and eccentric or asymmetric LV remodeling. Both afterload- and preload-related factors operate with additive and synergistic effects.

As a result myocardial hypertrophy induces activation of cellular apoptotic signals and activates metabolic pathways able to increase extracellular matrix production 'till to fibrosis [26, 27]. Fibrosis leads to a progressive impairment in contractility and a stiffening of the myocardial wall, leading to systolic and diastolic dysfunction, dilated cardiomyopathy and congestive heart failure [28]. Fibrosis also leads to disturbances of cardiac electrophysiology because of ventricular electrical conductance impairment and development re-entry pathways arrhythmias [17].

RAAS activation induces hyperaldosteronemia promoting cardiac fibrosis through generation of signals promoting profibrotic transforming growth factor production [21]. LVH can also be promoted by iron and/or erythropoietin [49] or by vitamin D deficiency [30]. Calciomimetics therapy can induce cardiac fibrosis regression without affecting left ventricular mass [31]. AV fistulas (AVFs) can contribute to LVH because of excess blood flow can contribute to LVH due to increased myocardial workload [14].

Arterial stiffness is mainly caused by increased collagen production and deposition with consequent increase in peripheral resistance due to vasoconstriction. Stiffness can also be caused by elevations in plasma sodium concentration (above 135 mMol/L) directly affecting vascular endothelium and nitric oxide release [32]. Modulation of plasma sodium concentrations during dialysis sessions can produce positive effects on blood pressure levels and left ventricular compliance [33].

Recent studies have pointed up their focus on novel biomarkers involved in the pathogenesis of LVH. One of these is represented by FGF23, member of fibroblast growth factors family primarly involved in CKD – MBD and secondary hyperparathyroidism.

Pathogenesis of CKD-MBD has always been ascribed to a decline in 1,25-dihydroxyvitamin D (1,25(OH)2D) levels leading to increases in serum parathyroid hormone (PTH) and subsequent alterations in calcium and phosphorus metabolism [34, 35]. Vitamin D deficiency, together with secondary hyperparathyroidism and hyperphosphatemia, was reported as a main factor contributing to high cardiovascular risks in CKD patients [36]. Discovery of fibroblast growth factor 23 changed what above described because of its role in secondary hyperparathyroidism pathophysiology. FGF23, at present time, represents earliest detected serum abnormality in patients with CKD – MBD [37] and FGF23 levels rises before any change in PTH,1,25(OH)2D, or serum phosphate levels [38]. FGF-23 is implicated in regulation,growth, and differentiation of cardiac myocytes holding paracrine functions in the kidneys because of its phosphaturic properties; it blocks vitamin D3 synthesis and inhibits proximal nephron reabsorption [39].

Serum levels of FGF23 increase gradually as kidney function decreases. FGF23 levels are often 2–5 times the normal levelduring the early and intermediate stages of CKD and can reach more than 200 times the normal level in cases of advanced renal failure [40]. First data about correlations between FGF23 levels and mortality were reported in 2008 when Gutierrez et al., evaluated FGF23 levels in over 400 hemodialysis starting patients. The increasedFGF23 levels at the initiation of dialysis were independently associated with significantly increased risk of subsequentmortality during the first year on dialysis [40].

Results of these observations were confirmed in two large longitudinal cohort studies in predialysis CKD patients. CRIC study enrolled 3879 CKD stage 2–4 patients with median follow-up of 3.5 years [41]; higher levels of FGF23 were associated independently with a greater risk of death. In post - hoc analysis of HOST study [42], a strong relation was found between higher FGF23 levels and higher risks of cardiovascular events and elevated C – terminal FGF23 was strongly associated with increased risk of acute myocardial infarction and lower extremity amputation.

Results of several clinical trials indicate a relation between FGF23 and LVH. In one of these 124 hemodialysis patients were evaluated for LVH and their respective FGF23 levels were independently associated with LVH [43]. Another study of 162 pre - dialysis CKD patients showed that FGF23 is independently associated with the left ventricular mass index and LVH [44].

Referring to CRIC study [32] higher C-terminal FGF23 levels were independently associated with reduced ejection fraction, greater left ventricular mass index and greater prevalence of both eccentric and concentric LVH [32].

Closely linked to CKD-MBD clinical features, several studies indicate a relationship between vitamin D, survival, vascular calcification and inflammation [45, 46] together with its central role in the regulation of bone mineral metabolism.

Vitamin D is also involved in the regulation of immune, cardiovascular and endocrine systems through the activation of the high-affinity nuclear vitamin D receptor (VDR).

Due to the relevant role of vitamin D in heart disease, the association between LVH and VDR gene polymorphisms has been recently investigated and it has been reported that the VDR BsmI gene polymorphism is involved in LVH in ESRD patients [47, 48] and independently related to LVH and LVH progression in dialysis patients and in stage IIIb CKD patients. The presence of BsmI mutated variant of VDR gene in ESRD patients has been proposed as a novel marker of disturbed vitamin D signaling pathway, determining consequently an increase in left ventricle mass (LVM) [48].

4. Clinical Consequences of Increased Left Ventricular (LV) Mass and Fibrosis in CKD and ESRD

As consequence of LVH, myocardial apoptosis and intermyocardial fibrosis, there is a decrease in myocardial capillary density, diastolic dysfunction (impaired diastolic filling of the ventricle to increased myocardial stiffness), systolic dysfunction and disturbances in intraventricular conduction, chamber dilation, and progressively more compensatory hypertrophy, dilation and dysfunction (uremic cardiomyopathy) [18]. Severity and persistence of LVH are strongly associated with mortality risk and cardiovascular events in CKD and in ESRD as reported by Zoccali [49] and London that found how a 10% decrease in LV mass translated into a 28% decrease in mortality risk from cardiovascular in a cohort of patients treated with hemodialysis [50]. Predictors of LVH regression included better control of systolic BP, a lower pulse wave velocity and rise in hemoglobin levels [50].

Despite of optimized risk factors' control (blood pressure, chronic ischemic heart disease and diabetes), sudden death often occurs in ESRD patients to underline that other factors (apart from coronary artery disease) have to been involved, such as LVH and myocardial fibrosis.

The presence of LVH almost doubled the risk of sudden cardiac death in the group of patients enrolled in the 4D trial [51]. Rising plasma levels of NT-pro-BNP have also been linked to sudden cardiac death in the 4D trial [51] together with metabolic (*e.g.,* hyperphosphatemia, hyperparathyroidism) and electrolyte (potassium, pH) alterations, sympathetic overactivity, autonomic nerve dysfunction, concomitant obstructive sleep apnea, acquired or hereditary QT interval prolongation, systolic and/or diastolic dysfunction, acute volume overload, and acute myocardial ischemia [17]. Autoptic studies in CKD patients show presence of diffuse inter-myocardiocyte fibrosis specific to the CKD patient heart, not observed in similarly hypertensive patients without kidney disease [52]. LVH is strongly associated with poor outcomes in patients both with and without CKD; longitudinal and cross-sectional studies of the "natural history" of LV mass in CKD points to an increase in prevalence of LVH as renal dysfunction develops [53].

Systolic hypertension and elevated pulse pressure are strongly associated with LVH in those patients with advanced CKD, suggesting that fluid overload and increased arterial stiffness play a role in LVH even before the start of dialysis therapy [53]. Positive response to LV mass reduction include younger age, lower pulse pressure, and higher GFR [54]. Persistent or progressing LVH is strongly associated with an increase in the risk of mortality and cardiovascular events including sudden cardiac death in ESRD patients [49]. Reduction in the degree of LVH can be achieved by fluid and BP control together with anemia control [55]. Foley found that improvements in LV mass and systolic function after one year initiation of dialysis therapy were associated with reduction rates of cardiac failure but not ischemic cardiac events and death [56].

Covic reported a regression of LV mass in hemodialysis patients associated with improvements in anemia, serum phosphate level, and calcium - phosphate product [57].

Marchais found increased diastolic and mean arterial pressures, higher cardiac index, higher heart rate, and increased stroke index in hyperphosphatemic *versus* normo-phosphatemic patients [58].

Higher plasma phosphate is associated with signs of diastolic dysfunction and myocardial fibrosis and it's accountable for facilitating LVH; so hyperphosphatemia might be an appropriate target of treatment [59].

In conclusion, LVH develops since early stages of CKD and it's quite common in patients on renal replacement therapy. LVH regresses in about 50% of hemodialysis patients as far as in patients on peritoneal dialysis treatment.

It's not actually clear if more aggressive dialysis treatment schedules could affect LVH development and regression although left ventricular mass reduction is clearly associated with better rates of cardiovascular morbidity and mortality [59].

5. Key Principles of LVH Management in CKD and ESRD Patients

Key principles of treatment of LVH in CKD patients are mainly based on anemia and blood pressure control, together with management of secondary hyperparathyroidism.

The impact of anemia therapy (with EPO) on LVH in CKD and/or ESRD has been examined in numerous randomized controlled trials but most of them have failed to show any beneficial effect on LVH of correction of hemoglobin levels to normal or near normal values.

Parfrey reported a meta – analysis of 15 trial and showed how LV mass was reduced by anemia correction only in those subjects who had severe anemia at baseline (below 10 g/dl) and who were treated to a lower target hemoglobin level (below 12 g/dl) [60]. Chen et al., [61]. compared the effects of epoetin alfa to darbopoetin on LVH in subjects with CKD. Both agents were equally effective in lowering LV mass. Correction of severe anemia (hemoglobin < 10 g/dl) with EPO seems to mitigate LVH [62], but use of EPO to elevate hemoglobin above 12 g/dl in subjects with less severe anemia seems to have no added benefits for reduction of LV mass.

Maintenance of systolic BP at normal levels (< 140 mmHg) would be predicted to have beneficial effects on the course of LVH in CKD and ESRD [63 – 65], as far as fluid volume management and maintenance of a near euvolemic state [66].

Correction of the diverse abnormalities of divalent ion metabolism in CKD and ESRD (including vitamin D deficiency, hyperphosphatemia, and hyperparathyroidism) may have beneficial effects on LVH but we have no clinical trials at disposal [67]. Patients receiving vitamin D therapy show lower frequency of cardiovascular events and improved survival in observational studies [67]. Several trials have showed how failure of LVH regress is associated with higher PTH levels (often intact PTH levels > 500 pg/ml) [57].

Another key point in the management of LVH is to better manage hemodialysis sessions and peritoneal dialysis exchanges. More frequent hemodialysis (including short-daily or long-nocturnal dialysis) has been suggested as a new paradigm of treatment [68 – 70] and observational studies have shown that more frequent and longer hemodialysis sessions are associated with lower prevalence of LVH [68 – 70].

As previously discussed, SCD is the most common cause of cardiovascular mortality in ESRD [71]. Small randomized controlled trials showed a reduction of sudden cardiac death from 10.4 to 3.4% with the use of carvedilol in ESRD patients with dilated cardiomyopathy [72], although more larger trials with β - blockers are needed. β-blocker therapy should routinely be used in CKD and ESRD patients with prior non fatal coronary artery ischemic events.

In table 1 there are summarized key management principles to prevent LVH progression in CKD patients.

6. Diagnosis and Assessment of LVH

Electrocardiography (ECG), 2D and 3D echocardiography (ECHO) (Figure 2 and Figure 3) and cardiac magnetic resonance (CMRI) (Figure 4) represent three next steps to quantify and estimate the degree of LVH.

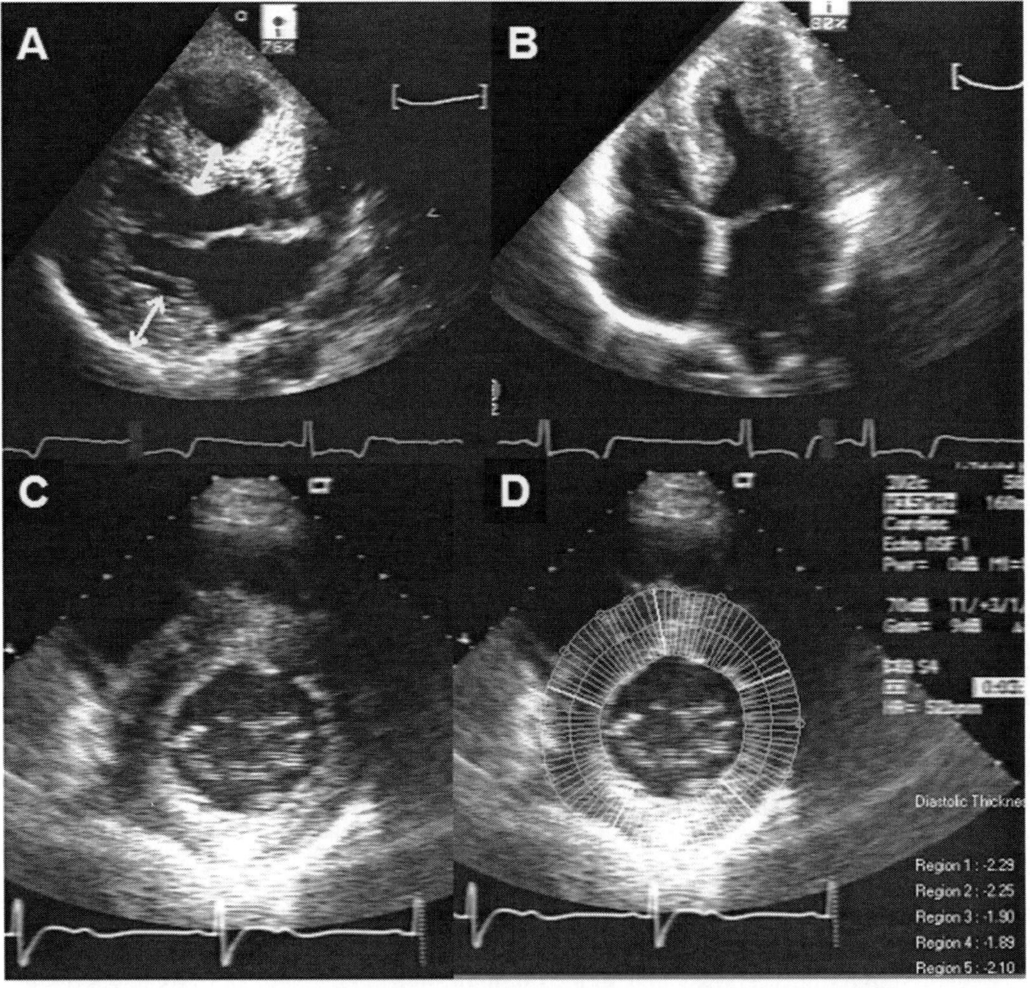

Figure 2. Two – dimensions echocardiography showing LVH in stage IIIb CKD patient.

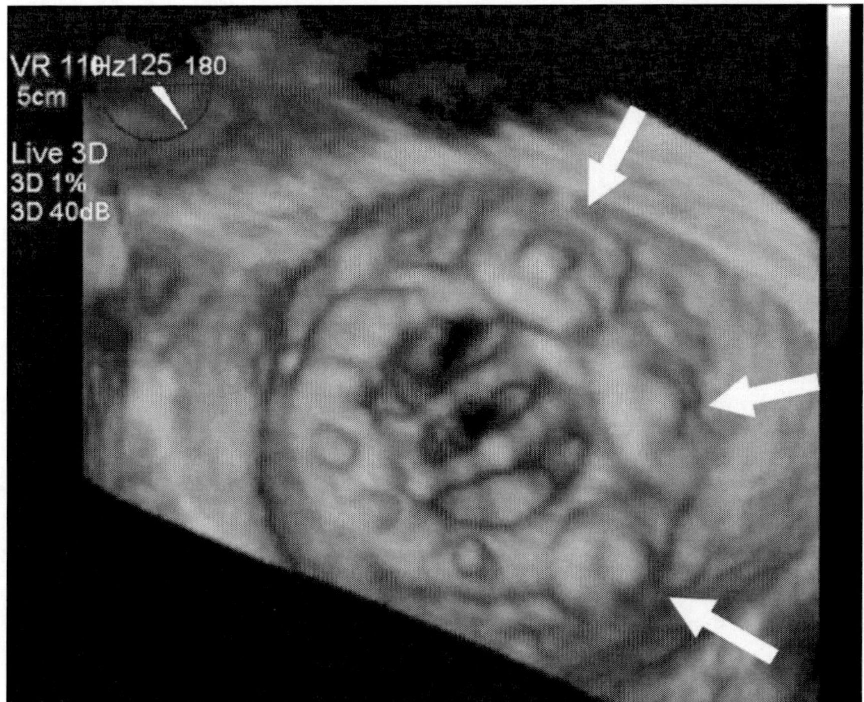

Figure 3. Three – dimensions echocardiography showing LVH in hemodialysis patient.

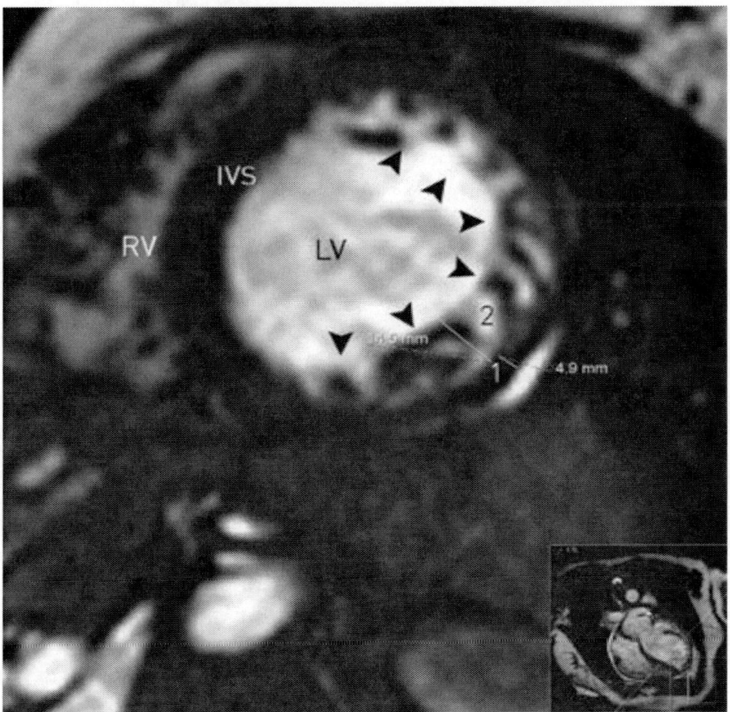

Figure 4. CMRI showing LVH in peritoneal dialysis patient.

Historically, electrocardiography (ECG) was first test employed to evaluate LVH because it's non – invasive, cheap and easily performed by nurses and physicians.

ECG is considered unsensitive ma quite specific method although criteria for ruling out LVH are not satisfactory [73].

On the other cardiac magnetic resonance represent the gold standard to evaluate left ventricular dimensions because it's accurate in defining left ventricular mass, volume and pattern of LVH (eccentric, concentric or asymmetric, and assessing fibrosis degree.

If we consider hemodialysis patients classical M – mode echocardiography often overestimates left ventricular mass compared to CMRI [74] but, on the other, CMRI cannot actually widespread employed due to costs and side effects as claustrophobia and presence of implantable devices in patients undergoing exam [75].

Because of clear limits of CMRI, ECHO is still established as main device to evaluate left ventricular mass in daily clinical practice although there are limitations in determination and quantification of LVH. ECHO accuracy depends on which technique is used, the timing of the test relative to the dialysis session, and the index used for "normalization" of the data generated. Therefore most LV mass estimates used linear measurements derived from M-mode ECHO that is subject to operator skill, patients' acoustic windows and other errors due to images' generation when we are in presence of an asymmetric left ventricular geometry [75, 76].

Variability in LV mass determination is credit to normalization's index adopted; because of left ventricular mass is proportional to body size, body surface is commonly used to make correction in classic studies and in clinical practice; so different cut – off values were used in different trials.

For example, Silverberg used a cut – off value of 125 g/m^2 [77], whereas Parfrey used values from Framingham study (132 g/m^2 for men and 100 g/m^2 for women) for diagnosis of LVH by ECHO [78]

Recent guidelines redefined normal values of LV mass as < 45 g/m-height [73, 76] for women and < 49 g/m height [73, 80] for men as defined by ECHO [79].

Two-dimensional (2-D) and three-dimensional (3-D) ECHO techniques have also been used to evaluate LV mass in CKD and ESRD but 2-D echocardiography is based on geometric assumptions and highly dependent of adequate endocardial and epicardial border definition of the LV. Real-time 3-D allows more precise assessment of LV mass, volume, and ejection fraction [79]. In comparison to other methods, 3-D echocardiography holds an accuracy quite close to CMRI [81].

In conclusion ECHO and CMRI may complementary in the evaluation of inter - myocardial fibrosis and diastolic dysfunction in CKD and ESRD [73] CMRI has the ability to detect and quantify the presence of myocardial fibrosis, as indicated by late gadolinium enhancement although it should be avoided in patients with late stages of CKD [82].

CMRI represent the best method for detecting and quantifying increased LV mass in CKD and ESRD but it's expensive and presents some practical restrictions while M-Mode or 2-D ECHO are widespread employed because they are cheaper and non – invasive techniques.

References

[1]   Ronco C: The cardiorenal syndrome: basis and common ground for a multidisciplinary patient-oriented therapy. *Cardiorenal Med* 2011; 1: 3–4.

[2]   Heywood JT, Fonarow GC, Costanzo MR, Mathur VS, Wigneswaran JR, Wynne J, ADHERE Scientific Advisory Committee and Investigators. High prevalence of renal dysfunction and its impact on outcome in 118,465 patients hospitalized with acute decompensated heart failure: A report from the ADHERE database. *J Card Fail* 13(6): 422-430, 2007

[3]   Garg AX, Clark WF, Haynes RB, House AA. Moderate renal insufficiency and the risk of cardiovascular mortality: Results from the NHANES I. *Kidney Int* 61(4): 1486-1494, 2002

[4]   Foley RN, Parfrey PS, Harnett JD, Kent GM, Murray DC, Barre PE. The prognostic importance of left ventricular geometry in uremic cardiomyopathy. *J Am Soc Nephrol* 5(12): 2024-2031, 1995

[5]   Harnett JD, Foley RN, Kent GM, Barre PE, Murray D, Parfrey PS. Congestive heart failure in dialysis patients: Prevalence, incidence, prognosis and risk factors. *Kidney Int* 47(3): 884-890, 1995

[6]   U.S. Renal Data System, USRDS 2012 Annual Data Report: Atlas of End-Stage Renal Disease in the United States, National Institutes of Health, National Institute of Diabetes and Digestive and Kidney Diseases, Bethesda, MD, 2012.

[7]   Tonelli M, Wiebe N, Culleton B, House A, Rabbat C, Fok M, McAlister F, Garg AX. Chronic kidney disease and mortality risk: A systematic review. *J Am Soc Nephrol* 17(7): 2034-2047, 2006

[8]   U.S. Renal Data System, USRDS 2009 Annual Data Report: Atlas of End-Stage Renal Disease in the United States, National Institutes of Health, National Institute of Diabetes and Digestive and Kidney Diseases, *Bethesda,* MD, 2009.

[9]   Go AS, Chertow GM, Fan D, McCulloch CE, Hsu CY. Chronic kidney disease and the risks of death, cardiovascular events, and hospitalization. *N Engl J Med* 351(13): 1296-1305, 2004

[10]   Shastri S, & Sarnak MJ. Cardiovascular disease and CKD: Core curriculum 2010. *Am J Kidney Dis* 56(2): 399-417, 2010

[11]   Stevens LA, Li S, Wang C, Huang C, Becker BN, Bomback AS, Brown WW, Burrows NR, Jurkovitz CT, McFarlane SI, Norris KC, Shlipak M, Whaley-Connell AT, Chen SC, Bakris GL, McCullough PA. Prevalence of CKD and comorbid illness in elderly patients in the united states: Results from the kidney early evaluation program (KEEP). *Am J Kidney Dis* 55(3 Suppl 2): S23-33, 2010

[12]   Bansal N, Keane M, Delafontaine P, Dries D, Foster E, Gadegbeku CA, Go AS, Hamm LL, Kusek JW, Ojo AO, Rahman M, Tao K, Wright JT, Xie D, Hsu CY, CRIC Study Investigators. A longitudinal study of left ventricular function and structure from CKD to ESRD: The CRIC study. *Clin J Am Soc Nephrol* 8(3): 355-362, 2013

[13]   Kottgen A, Russell SD, Loehr LR, Crainiceanu CM, Rosamond WD, Chang PP, Chambless LE, Coresh J. Reduced kidney function as a risk factor for incident heart failure: The atherosclerosis risk in communities (ARIC) study. *J Am Soc Nephrol* 18(4): 1307-1315, 2007

[14] Di Lullo L, Floccari F, Polito P: Right ventricular diastolic function in dialysis patients could be affected by vascular access. *Nephron Clin Pract* 2011; 118:c258–c262.

[15] Bologa RM, Levine DM, Parker TS, et al., Interleukin-6 predicts hypoalbuminemia, hypocholesterolemia, and mortality in hemodialysis patients. *Am J Kidney Dis* 32(1):107-114, 1998

[16] Parikh SV, de Lemos JA: Biomarkers in cardiovascular disease: integrating pathophysiology into clinical practice. *Am J Med Sci* 332(4):186-197, 2006

[17] Ritz E, Wanner C: The challenge of sudden death in dialysis patients. *Clin J Am Soc Nephrol* 3: 920-929, 2008

[18] Gross ML, Ritz E: Hypertrophy and fibrosis in the cardiomyopathy of uremia – beyond coronary heart disease. *Semin Dial* 21:308 – 318, 2008

[19] Ritz E: Left ventricular hypertrophy in renal disease: beyond preload and afterload. *Kidney Int* 75: 771–773, 2009

[20] Mominadam S et al., Interdialytic blood pressure obtained by ambulatory blood pressure measurement and left ventricular structure in hypertensive hemodialysis patients. *Hemodial Int* 12: 322–327, 2008

[21] Steigerwalt S, Zafar A, Mesiha N, Gardin J, Provenzano R: Role of aldosterone in left ventricular hypertrophy among African – American patients with end – stage renal disease on hemodialysis. *Am J Nephrol* 27: 159–163, 2007

[22] Xu X, Hu X, Zhang P, Zhao L, Wessale JL, Bache RJ, Chen Y: Xantine oxidase inhibition with febuxostat attenuates systolic overload-induced left ventricular hypertrophy and dysfunction in mice. *J Card Fail* 14: 746–753, 2008

[23] Hsu S, Nagayama T, Koitabashi N, Zhang M, Zhou L et al., Phosphodiesterase-5 inhibition blocks pressure overload-induced cardiac hypertrophy independent of the calcineurin pathway. *Cardiovasc Res* 81: 301–309, 2009

[24] Martin LC, Franco RJ, Gavras I, Matsubara BB, Garcia S, Caramori JT, Barretti BB, Balbi AR, Barsanti R, Padovani C, Gavras H: Association between hypervolemia and ventricular hypertrophy in hemodialysis patients. *Am J Hypertens* 17: 1163–1169, 2004

[25] McRae JM, Levin A, Belenkie I: The cardiovascular effects of arteriovenous fistulas in chronic kidney disease. A cause for concern ? *Semin Dial* 19: 349–352, 2006

[26] Nishida K, Kyoi S, Yamaguchi O, Sadoshima J, Otsu K: The role of autophagy in the heart. *Cell Death Differ* 16: 31–38, 2009

[27] Dorm GW 2nd: Apoptotic and non – apoptotic programmed cardiomyocyte death in ventricular remodeling. *Cardiovasc Res* 81: 465-473, 2009

[28] Zoccali C, Benedetto FA, Tripepi G, Mallamaci F: Cardiac consequences of hypertension in hemodialysis patients. *Semin Dial* 17: 299–303, 2004

[29] Sakurabayashi T, Miyazaki S, Yuasa Y, Sakai S, Suzuki M, Takahashi S, Hirasawa Y: L- carnitine supplementation decreases the left ventricular mass in patients undergoing hemodialysis. *Circ J* 72: 926–931, 2008

[30] Strozecki P et al., Parathormon, calcium, phosphorus and left ventricular structure and function in normotensive hemodialysis patients. *Ren Fail* 23: 115–126, 2001

[31] Koleganova N, Piecha G, Ritz E, Bekeredjian R, Schirmacher P, Schmitt CP, Gross ML: Interstitial fibrosis and microvascular disease of the heart in uremia: amelioration by a calciomimetic. *Lab Invest* 89: 520–530, 2009

[32] Oberleithner H, Riethmuller C, Schillers H, Mac Gregor GA, de Wardener HE, Hausberg M: Plasma sodium-stiffens vascular endothelium and reduces nitric oxide release. *Proc Natl Acad Sci U S A* 104: 16281–16286, 2007

[33] De Paula FM, Peixoto AJ, Pinto LV, Dorigo D, Patricio PJ, Santos SF: Clinical consequences of an individualized dialysate sodium prescription in hemodialysis patients. *Kidney Int* 66: 1232–1238, 2004

[34] Moe S, Drueke T, Cunningham J: Definition, evaluation and classification of renal osteodistrophy: a position statement from Kidney Disease Improving Global Outcome (KDIGO). *Kidney Int,* vol. 69, no. 11, pp. 1945–1953, 2006

[35] Moe S, Drueke TB, Block A et al., KDIGO clinical practice guideline for the diagnosis, evaluation, prevention and treatment of chronic kidney disease-mineral and bone disorder (CKD-MBD). *Kidney Int* 113; S1 – S130, 2009

[36] Burhiya R, Li S, Chen S, Mc Cullough PA, Bakris GL: Plasma parathyroid hormone level and prevalent cardiovascular disease in CKD stages 3 and 4: an analysis from the Kidney Early Evaluation Program (KEEP). *Am Journal of Kidney Disease* 53(4): S3-S10, 2009

[37] Evenepoel P, Meijers B, Viaene L et al., Fibroblast growth factor-23 in early chronic kidney disease: additional support in favor of a phosphate-centric paradigm for the pathogenesis of secondary hyperparathyroidism. *Clin Journal of Am Society of Nephrology* 5 (7): 1268-1276, 2010

[38] Isakova T, Wahl P, Vargas GS: : Fibroblast growth factor-23 is elevated before parathyroid hormone and phosphate in chronic kidney disease. *Kidney Int* 79 (12): 1370-1378, 2011

[39] Faul C, Amaral AP, Oskouei B et al., FGF23 induces left ventricular hyperthrophy. *J Clin Invest* 12: 4393 – 4408, 2011

[40] Gutierrez OM, Mannstadt M, Isakova T et al., Fibroblast growth factor 23 and mortality among patients undergoing hemodialysis. *The New England Journal of Medicine*, 359 (6): 584-592, 2008

[41] Isakova T, Xie H, Yang W: Fibroblast growth factor 23 and risks of mortality and end – stage renal disease in patients with chronic kidney disease. *Journal of the American Medical Association* 305 (23): 2432-2439, 2011

[42] Liu X, Xie R, Liu S: Rat parathyroid hormone 1–34 signals through the MEK/ERK pathway to induce cardiac hyper- trophy. *J Int Med Res* 36: 942–950, 2008

[43] Moon KH, Song IS, Yang WS, Shin YT, Kim SB, Song JK, Park JS: Hypoalbuminemia as a risk factor for progressive left-ventricular hypertrophy in hemodialysis patients. *Am J Nephrol* 20: 396 – 401, 2000

[44] Chmielewski M, Carrero JJ, Stenvinkel P, Lindholm B: Metabolic abnormalities in chronic kidney disease that contribute to cardiovascular disease, and nutritional initiatives that may diminish the risk. *Curr Opin Lipidol* 20: 3–9, 2009

[45] Wolf M, Shah A, Gutierrez O, Ankers E, Monroy M, Tamez H, Steele D, Chang Y. Camargo CA Jr, Tonelli M, Thadhani R: Vitamin D levels and early mortality among incident hemodialysis patients. *Kidney Int.* 2007, *72*, 1004–1013.

[46] Mehrotra R, Kermah D, Budoff M, Salusky IB, Mao SS, Gao YL, Takasu J, Adler S, Norris K: Hypovitaminosis D in chronic kidney disease. *Clin. J. Am. Soc. Nephrol.* 2008, *3*, 1144–1151.

[47] Testa A, Mallamaci F, Benedetto F, Pisano A, Tripepi G, Malatino L, Thadhani R, Zoccali C: Vitamin D Receptor (VDR) Gene Polymorphism Is Associated With Left Ventricular (LV) Mass and Predicts Left Ventricular Hypertrophy (LVH) Progression in End-Stage Renal Disease (ESRD) Patients. *J. Bone Miner. Res.* 2010, 25, 313–319.

[48] El-Shehaby AM, El-Khatib MM, Marzouk S, Battah AA: Relationship of BsmI polymorphism of vitamin D receptor gene with left ventricular hypertrophy and atherosclerosis in hemodialysis patients. *Scand J. Clin. Lab. Investig.* 2013, 73, 75–81.

[49] Zoccali C, Benedetto FA, Mallamaci F, Tripepi G, Giacone G, Stancanelli B, Cataliotti A, Malatino LS: Left ventricular mass monitoring in the follow-up of dialysis patients: Prognostic value of left ventricular hypertrophy progres- sion. *Kidney Int* 65: 1492–1498, 2004

[50] London GM, Pannier B, Guerin AP, Blacher J, Marchais SJ, Darne B, Metivier F, Adda H, Safar ME: Alterations of left ventricular hypertrophy in and survival of patients receiv- ing hemodialysis: follow-up of an interventional study. *J Am Soc Nephrol* 12: 2759 –2767, 2001

[51] Krane V, Winkler K, Drechsler C, Lilienthal J, Marz W, Wanner C: Effect of atorvastatin on inflammation and out- come in patients with type 2 diabetes mellitus on hemodi- alysis. *Kidney Int* 74: 1461–1467, 2008

[52] Aoki J, Ikari Y, Nakajima H, Mori M, Sugimoto T, Hatori M, Tanimoto S, Amiya E, Hara K: Clinical and pathologic characteristics of dilated cardiomyopathy in hemodialysis patients. *Kidney Int* 67: 333–340, 2005

[53] Paoletti E, Bellino D, Cassottana P, Rolla D, Cannella G: Left ventricular hypertrophy in nondiabetic predialysis CKD. *Am J Kidney Dis* 46: 320 –327, 2005

[54] McMahon LP, Roger SD, Levin A: Development, preven- tion, and potential reversal of left ventricular hypertrophy in chronic kidney disease. *J Am Soc Nephrol* 15: 1640 – 1647, 2004

[55] Culleton BF, Walsh M, Klarenbach SW, Mortis G, Scott- Douglas N, Quinn RR, Tonelli M, Donnelly S, Friedrich MG, Kumar A, Mahallati H, Hemmelgarn BR, Manns BJ: Effect of frequent nocturnal hemodialysis vs conventional hemodialysis on left ventricular mass and quality of life: A randomized controlled trial. *JAMA* 298: 1291– 1299, 2007

[56] Foley RN, Parfrey PS, Kent GM, Harnett JD, Murray DC, Barre PE: Serial change in echocardiographic parameters and cardiac failure in end-stage renal disease. *J Am Soc Nephrol* 11: 912–916, 2000

[57] Covic A, Mardare NG, Ardeleanu S, Prisada O, Gusbeth- Tatomir P, Goldsmith DJ: Serial echocardiographic changes in patients on hemodialysis: An evaluation of guideline implementation. *J Nephrol* 19: 783–793, 2006

[58] Marchais SJ, Metivier F, Guerin AP, London GM: Associ- ation of hyperphosphataemia with haemodynamic distur- bances in end-stage renal disease. *Nephrol Dial Transplant* 14: 2178 –2183, 1999

[59] Galetta F, Cupisti A, Franzoni F, Femia FR, Rossi M, Bar- sotti G, Santoro G: Left ventricular function and calcium phosphate plasma levels in uraemic patients. *J Intern Med* 258: 378 –384, 2005

[60] Parfrey PS, Lauve M, Latremouille-Viau D, Lefebvre P: Erythropoietin therapy and left ventricular mass index in CKD and ESRD patients: A meta-analysis. *Clin J Am Soc Nephrol* 4: 755–762, 2009

Clinical Definition of LVH

h several electrocardiographic (ECG) criteria for the identification of LVH are
dditional investigations (notably transthoracic echocardiography (echo)) are
quired due to the lack of sensitivity and specificity of ECG. The European
of Echocardiography definition of LVH includes the demonstration of
lar septum and/or posterior wall thickness in end-diastole of ≥13mm. [2] In
hocardiography can interrogate valve function and characterize LVH as
uniform mechanism e.g., LV pressure overload, myocardial infiltration), or
., asymmetrical septal hypertrophy in hypertrophic cardiomyopathy (HCM)).

actical Approach to Evaluation of LVH

identification of LVH, a practical approach to its further assessment includes a
w with targeted investigations aimed firstly to exclude common causes which are
. Thereafter evaluation involves a systematic approach to exclude less common
timately instigate tailored individual treatment strategy.

Causes of LVH

causes of LVH are hypertension, aortic stenosis and obesity. Physiological
e from high level of endurance training such as athletic heart. Other rarer but
ses include: sarcomere protein disease (e.g., hypertrophic cardiomyopathy),
nfiltration (e.g., amyloidosis, Haemo-chromatosis), left ventricular non
metabolic disorders (e.g., Fabry's disease, Pompe disease, Danon disease,
diomyopathy, primary carnitine deficiency), mitochondrial myopathies (e.g.,
syndrome, MERFF syndrome, MELAS syndrome), syndromic conditions (e.g.,
ome, Friedreich's ataxia).

mmarises the causes of LVH and their diagnostic pointers. Disorders causing
with LVH are arranged in a pathological hierarchical manner with common
earing first, followed by rarities. Many heart muscle disorders presenting with
to inherited mutations in genes encoding contractile proteins of the cardiac
tabolic pathways, or mitochondrial proteins. [3] Hypertrophic cardiomyopathy
nest inherited cardiac condition and an important cause of (potentially
udden arrhythmic death. As such it is placed high in table and should be
y in the diagnostic work-up of unexplained LVH.

Treatment of LVH

of the underlying causes is essential and each of the important reversible
ssed as follows.

[61] Chen HH, Tarng DC, Lee KF, Wu CY, Chen YC: Epoetin alfa and darbepoetin alfa: Effects on ventricular hypertro- phy in patients with chronic kidney disease. *J Nephrol* 21: 543–549, 2008

[62] Ayus JC, Go AS, Valderrabano F, Verde E, de Vinuesa SG, Achinger SG, Lorenzo V, Arieff AI, Luno J: Effects of erythropoietin on left ventricular hypertrophy in adults with severe chronic renal failure and hemoglobin 10 g/dL. *Kidney Int* 68: 788 –795, 2005

[63] Mattioli AV, Zennaro M, Bonatti S, Bonetti L, Mattioli G: Regression of left ventricular hypertrophy and improve- ment of diastolic function in hypertensive patients treated with telmisartan. *Int J Cardiol* 97: 383–388, 2004

[64] Devereux RB, Palmieri V, Liu JE, Wachtell K, Bella JN, Boman K, Gerdts E, Nieminen MS, Papademetriou V, Dahlof B: Progressive hypertrophy regression with sus- tained pressure reduction in hypertension: The Losartan Intervention For Endpoint Reduction study. *J Hypertens* 20: 1445–1450, 2002

[65] Jula AM, Karanko HM: Effects on left ventricular hyper- trophy of long-term nonpharmacological treatment with sodium restriction in mild-to-moderate essential hyperten- sion. *Circulation* 89: 1023–1031, 1994

[66] Charra B, Chazot C: Volume control, blood pressure and cardiovascular function. Lessons from hemodialysis treat- ment. *Nephron Physiol* 93: 94 –101, 2003

[67] Achinger SG, Ayus JC: The role of vitamin D in left ven- tricular hypertrophy and cardiac function. *Kidney Int* 68: Suppl: S37–S42, 2005

[68] Ly J, Chan CT: Impact of augmenting dialysis frequency and duration on cardiovascular function. *ASAIO J* 52: e11– e14, 2006

[69] Fagugli RM, Pasini P, Pasticci F, Ciao G, Cicconi B, Buon- cristiani U: Effects of short daily hemodialysis and ex- tended standard hemodialysis on blood pressure and car- diac hypertrophy: A comparative study. *J Nephrol* 19: 77– 83, 2006

[70] Weinreich T, De los Rios T, Gauly A, Passlick-Deetjen J: Effects of an increase in time vs. frequency on cardiovas- cular parameters in chronic hemodialysis patients. *Clin Nephrol* 66: 433– 439, 2006

[71] Kong CH, Farrington K: Determinants of left ventricular hypertrophy and its progression in high-flux haemodialy- sis. *Blood Purif* 21: 163–169, 2003

[72] Cice G, Ferrara L, D'Andrea A, D'Isa S, Di Benedetto A, Cittadini A, Russo PE, Golino P, Calabro R: Carvedilol increases two-year survivalin dialysis patients with dilated cardiomyopathy: A prospective, placebo-controlled trial. *J Am Coll Cardiol* 41: 1438 –1444, 2003

[73] Pewsner D, Juni P, Egger M, Battaglia M, Sundstrom J, Bachmann LM: Accuracy of electrocardiography in diag- nosis of left ventricular hypertrophy in arterial hyperten- sion: systematic review. *BMJ* 335: 711, 2007

[74] Stewart GA, Foster J, Cowan M, Rooney E, McDonagh T, Dargie HJ, Rodger RS, Jardine AG: Echocardiography overestimates left ventricular mass in hemodialysis patients relative to magnetic resonance imaging. *Kidney Int* 56: 2248 –2253, 1999

[75] Mark PB, Patel RK, Jardine AG: Are we overestimating left ventricular abnormalities in end-stage renal disease? *Nephrol Dial Transplant* 22: 1815–1819, 2007

[76] Zoccali C, Benedetto FA, Mallamaci F, Tripepi G, Giacone G, Cataliotti A, Seminara G, Stancanelli B, Malatino LS: Prognostic impact of the indexation of left ventricular mass in patients undergoing dialysis. *J Am Soc Nephrol* 12: 2768 – 2774, 2001

[77] Silberberg JS, Barre PE, Prichard SS, Sniderman AD: Im- pact of left ventricular hypertrophy on survival in end- stage renal disease. *Kidney Int* 36: 286 –290, 1989

[78] Parfrey PS, Foley RN, Harnett JD, Kent GM, Murray DC, Barre PE: Outcome and risk factors for left ventricular disorders in chronic uraemia. *Nephrol Dial Transplant* 11: 1277–1285, 1996

[79] Lang RM, Bierig M, Devereux RB, Flachskampf FA, Foster E, Pellikka PA, Picard MH, Roman MJ, Seward J, Shane- wise JS, Solomon SD, Spencer KT, Sutton MS, Stewart WJ: Recommendations for chamber quantification: a report from the American Society of Echocardiography's Guide- lines and Standards Committee and the Chamber Quanti- fication Writing Group, developed in conjunction with the European Association of Echocardiography, a branch of the European Society of Cardiology. *J Am Soc Echocardiogr* 18: 1440 –1463, 2005

[80] Ritz E, Bommer J: Cardiovascular problems on hemo- dialysis: current deficits and potential improvement. *Clin J Am Soc Nephrol* 4: S71–S78, 2009

[81] Takeuchi M, Nishikage T, Mor-Avi V, Sugeng L, Weinert L, Nakai H, Salgo IS, Gerard O, Lang RM: Measurement of left ventricular mass by real-time three-dimensional echo- cardiography: Validation against magnetic resonance and comparison with two-dimensional and m-mode measure- ments. *J Am Soc Echocardiogr* 21: 1001–1005, 2008

[82] Kribben A, Witzke O, Hillen U, Barkhausen J, Daul AE, Erbel R: Nephrogenic systemic fibrosis: Pathogenesis, di- agnosis, and therapy. *J Am Coll Cardiol* 53: 1621– 1628, 2009

In: Left Ventricular Hypertrophy (LVH)
Editor: Richard T. Matthews   © 201

Clinical Evaluation of Left Hypertrophy

Eveline Lee and Zaheer*
University Hospital of Wales, Ca

Abstract

Left ventricular hypertrophy (LVH) is prevalent Although the relative risk of cardiovascular mortality ventricular mass, many underlying causes are reversible i

We discuss the clinical definition and diagnostic crit factors and treatment. A pragmatic systematic appr assessment and investigations of the common (hyper obesity, athletic heart) and rare (inherited, infiltrative a underlying causes of LVH.

Introduction

Left ventricular hypertrophy (LVH) is prevalent a Framingham Heart Study [1], it is present in 15-20% o 50g/m2 of left ventricular mass, there is an increase in re 1.73 in men and 2.12 in women. Nonetheless many of reversible if timely investigation and treatment are instiga

---

* E-mail: LeeE4@cardiff.ac.uk.

[61] Chen HH, Tarng DC, Lee KF, Wu CY, Chen YC: Epoetin alfa and darbepoetin alfa: Effects on ventricular hypertro- phy in patients with chronic kidney disease. *J Nephrol* 21: 543–549, 2008

[62] Ayus JC, Go AS, Valderrabano F, Verde E, de Vinuesa SG, Achinger SG, Lorenzo V, Arieff AI, Luno J: Effects of erythropoietin on left ventricular hypertrophy in adults with severe chronic renal failure and hemoglobin 10 g/dL. *Kidney Int* 68: 788 –795, 2005

[63] Mattioli AV, Zennaro M, Bonatti S, Bonetti L, Mattioli G: Regression of left ventricular hypertrophy and improve- ment of diastolic function in hypertensive patients treated with telmisartan. *Int J Cardiol* 97: 383–388, 2004

[64] Devereux RB, Palmieri V, Liu JE, Wachtell K, Bella JN, Boman K, Gerdts E, Nieminen MS, Papademetriou V, Dahlof B: Progressive hypertrophy regression with sus- tained pressure reduction in hypertension: The Losartan Intervention For Endpoint Reduction study. *J Hypertens* 20: 1445–1450, 2002

[65] Jula AM, Karanko HM: Effects on left ventricular hyper- trophy of long-term nonpharmacological treatment with sodium restriction in mild-to-moderate essential hyperten- sion. *Circulation* 89: 1023–1031, 1994

[66] Charra B, Chazot C: Volume control, blood pressure and cardiovascular function. Lessons from hemodialysis treat- ment. *Nephron Physiol* 93: 94 –101, 2003

[67] Achinger SG, Ayus JC: The role of vitamin D in left ven- tricular hypertrophy and cardiac function. *Kidney Int* 68: Suppl: S37–S42, 2005

[68] Ly J, Chan CT: Impact of augmenting dialysis frequency and duration on cardiovascular function. *ASAIO J* 52: e11– e14, 2006

[69] Fagugli RM, Pasini P, Pasticci F, Ciao G, Cicconi B, Buon- cristiani U: Effects of short daily hemodialysis and ex- tended standard hemodialysis on blood pressure and car- diac hypertrophy: A comparative study. *J Nephrol* 19: 77– 83, 2006

[70] Weinreich T, De los Rios T, Gauly A, Passlick-Deetjen J: Effects of an increase in time vs. frequency on cardiovas- cular parameters in chronic hemodialysis patients. *Clin Nephrol* 66: 433– 439, 2006

[71] Kong CH, Farrington K: Determinants of left ventricular hypertrophy and its progression in high-flux haemodialy- sis. *Blood Purif* 21: 163–169, 2003

[72] Cice G, Ferrara L, D'Andrea A, D'Isa S, Di Benedetto A, Cittadini A, Russo PE, Golino P, Calabro R: Carvedilol increases two-year survivalin dialysis patients with dilated cardiomyopathy: A prospective, placebo-controlled trial. *J Am Coll Cardiol* 41: 1438 –1444, 2003

[73] Pewsner D, Juni P, Egger M, Battaglia M, Sundstrom J, Bachmann LM: Accuracy of electrocardiography in diag- nosis of left ventricular hypertrophy in arterial hyperten- sion: systematic review. *BMJ* 335: 711, 2007

[74] Stewart GA, Foster J, Cowan M, Rooney E, McDonagh T, Dargie HJ, Rodger RS, Jardine AG: Echocardiography overestimates left ventricular mass in hemodialysis patients relative to magnetic resonance imaging. *Kidney Int* 56: 2248 –2253, 1999

[75] Mark PB, Patel RK, Jardine AG: Are we overestimating left ventricular abnormalities in cnd-stage renal disease? *Nephrol Dial Transplant* 22: 1815–1819, 2007

[76] Zoccali C, Benedetto FA, Mallamaci F, Tripepi G, Giacone G, Cataliotti A, Seminara G, Stancanelli B, Malatino LS: Prognostic impact of the indexation of left ventricular mass in patients undergoing dialysis. *J Am Soc Nephrol* 12: 2768 – 2774, 2001

[77] Silberberg JS, Barre PE, Prichard SS, Sniderman AD: Im- pact of left ventricular hypertrophy on survival in end- stage renal disease. *Kidney Int* 36: 286 –290, 1989

[78] Parfrey PS, Foley RN, Harnett JD, Kent GM, Murray DC, Barre PE: Outcome and risk factors for left ventricular disorders in chronic uraemia. *Nephrol Dial Transplant* 11: 1277–1285, 1996

[79] Lang RM, Bierig M, Devereux RB, Flachskampf FA, Foster E, Pellikka PA, Picard MH, Roman MJ, Seward J, Shane- wise JS, Solomon SD, Spencer KT, Sutton MS, Stewart WJ: Recommendations for chamber quantification: a report from the American Society of Echocardiography's Guide- lines and Standards Committee and the Chamber Quanti- fication Writing Group, developed in conjunction with the European Association of Echocardiography, a branch of the European Society of Cardiology. *J Am Soc Echocardiogr* 18: 1440 –1463, 2005

[80] Ritz E, Bommer J: Cardiovascular problems on hemo- dialysis: current deficits and potential improvement. *Clin J Am Soc Nephrol* 4: S71–S78, 2009

[81] Takeuchi M, Nishikage T, Mor-Avi V, Sugeng L, Weinert L, Nakai H, Salgo IS, Gerard O, Lang RM: Measurement of left ventricular mass by real-time three-dimensional echo- cardiography: Validation against magnetic resonance and comparison with two-dimensional and m-mode measure- ments. *J Am Soc Echocardiogr* 21: 1001–1005, 2008

[82] Kribben A, Witzke O, Hillen U, Barkhausen J, Daul AE, Erbel R: Nephrogenic systemic fibrosis: Pathogenesis, di- agnosis, and therapy. *J Am Coll Cardiol* 53: 1621– 1628, 2009

In: Left Ventricular Hypertrophy (LVH)
Editor: Richard T. Matthews

ISBN: 978-1-63463-022-1
© 2015 Nova Science Publishers, Inc.

Chapter 4

Clinical Evaluation of Left Ventricular Hypertrophy

Eveline Lee and *Zaheer Yosuef*
University Hospital of Wales, Cardiff, UK

Abstract

Left ventricular hypertrophy (LVH) is prevalent and carries poor prognosis. Although the relative risk of cardiovascular mortality increases with incremental left ventricular mass, many underlying causes are reversible if timely treatment is instigated.

We discuss the clinical definition and diagnostic criteria of LVH, its prevalence, risk factors and treatment. A pragmatic systematic approach is adopted for targeted assessment and investigations of the common (hypertension, valvular heart disease, obesity, athletic heart) and rare (inherited, infiltrative and metabolic cardiomyopathies) underlying causes of LVH.

Introduction

Left ventricular hypertrophy (LVH) is prevalent and carries poor prognosis. In the Framingham Heart Study [1], it is present in 15-20% of adults and for every incremental 50g/m2 of left ventricular mass, there is an increase in relative risk of cardiovascular death of 1.73 in men and 2.12 in women. Nonetheless many of the underlying causes of LVH are reversible if timely investigation and treatment are instigated.

---

* E-mail: LeeE4@cardiff.ac.uk.

Clinical Definition of LVH

Although several electrocardiographic (ECG) criteria for the identification of LVH are available, additional investigations (notably transthoracic echocardiography (echo)) are invariably required due to the lack of sensitivity and specificity of ECG. The European Association of Echocardiography definition of LVH includes the demonstration of interventricular septum and/or posterior wall thickness in end-diastole of $\geq$13mm. [2] In addition, echocardiography can interrogate valve function and characterize LVH as concentric (uniform mechanism e.g., LV pressure overload, myocardial infiltration), or eccentric (e.g., asymmetrical septal hypertrophy in hypertrophic cardiomyopathy (HCM)).

Practical Approach to Evaluation of LVH

After the identification of LVH, a practical approach to its further assessment includes a clinical review with targeted investigations aimed firstly to exclude common causes which are often treatable. Thereafter evaluation involves a systematic approach to exclude less common causes and ultimately instigate tailored individual treatment strategy.

Causes of LVH

Common causes of LVH are hypertension, aortic stenosis and obesity. Physiological LVH can arise from high level of endurance training such as athletic heart. Other rarer but important causes include: sarcomere protein disease (e.g., hypertrophic cardiomyopathy), myocardial infiltration (e.g., amyloidosis, Haemo-chromatosis), left ventricular non compaction, metabolic disorders (e.g., Fabry's disease, Pompe disease, Danon disease, PRKAG2 cardiomyopathy, primary carnitine deficiency), mitochondrial myopathies (e.g., Kearns-Sayra syndrome, MERFF syndrome, MELAS syndrome), syndromic conditions (e.g., Noonan syndrome, Friedreich's ataxia).

Table 1 summarises the causes of LVH and their diagnostic pointers. Disorders causing or associated with LVH are arranged in a pathological hierarchical manner with common conditions appearing first, followed by rarities. Many heart muscle disorders presenting with LVH are due to inherited mutations in genes encoding contractile proteins of the cardiac sarcomere, metabolic pathways, or mitochondrial proteins. [3] Hypertrophic cardiomyopathy is the commonest inherited cardiac condition and an important cause of (potentially preventable) sudden arrhythmic death. As such it is placed high in table and should be considered early in the diagnostic work-up of unexplained LVH.

Treatment of LVH

Treatment of the underlying causes is essential and each of the important reversible causes is discussed as follows.

1. **Hypertension**

   Stratify overall cardiovascular risks, exclude secondary hypertension, employ lifestyle modification (including dietary salt restriction, weight reduction, exercise promotion, smoking cessation, increase intake of fruit and vegetables) , treat to target blood pressure, often requiring >2 agents. [4]

2. **Aortic stenosis**

   Use multi-modalities cardiac imaging for comprehensive assessment of severity. Multidisciplinary team (MDT) directed management for individually tailored management plan. Severe valve stenosis should be replaced surgically unless surgery is deemed unsuitable or high risk by MDT, in which case transcatheter aortic valve implantation (TAVI) may be an alternative. [5]

3. **Obesity**

   Life style modification, weight control, consider drug treatment, refer for specialist assessment for consideration of bariatric intervention. [6]

4. **Hypertrophic cardiomyopathy**

   Early risk stratification (e.g., exercise tolerance test, family history, previous aborted sudden cardiac death) to identify high risk patients and consider implantable cardiac defibrillator. Offer longitudinal follow up to individuals affected genetically but without phenotype. Use medications such as beta blockers, verapamil and disopyramide to reduce outflow tract gradient and control symptoms. Consider surgical myectomy for those with refractory outflow tract obstruction symptoms, alternatives to surgery include dual chamber pacing and alcohol septal ablation. [7]

5. **Amyloidosis**

   Cross specialty investigations to determine the form of amyloid. Supportive therapy of all types of amyloid such as diuretics for heart failure symptoms, pleural tap or pleurodesis for recurrent pleural effusions/pleural Amyloidosis, consider anticoagulation if atrial fibrillation present. Anti plasma cell therapy to reduce paraprotein production suitable for AL Amyloidosis, chemotherapy/bone marrow transplant/cardiac transplant may be suitable in selected subjects. [8]

6. **Haemo-chromatosis**

   Early identification and pre emptive treatment (venesection) guided by levels of haemotocrit/haemoglobin and serum ferritin. Avoid vitamin C and consider iron chelation therapy. [9]

7. **Fabry's disease**

   Once established, end organ damage is irreversible; therefore early diagnosis and supportive therapy are essential. Enzyme replacement therapy (e.g., agalsidase alpha and agalsidase beta) reduces clinical events, promotes LV remodelling, improves cardiac function and exercise tolerance. [10-12]

Conclusion

LVH remains a common pathology which requires exhaustive characterisation. In most cases, LVH may be attributable to hypertension, vale disease, or obesity. It is important, however, not to miss potentially treatable conditions and initiate the appropriate treatment early. We discussed a systematic approach to investigations of common and important underlying causes.

Table 1. Causes of LVH, with clinical characteristics and diagnostic pointers

	Condition	Clinical Pearls	Diagnostic Pointers
Common causes	Hypertension	~15% secondary cause Fundoscopic changes Lost nocturnal dip on 24hour recording 60%: ≥2 hypotensives needed to achieve control	ECG: LVH(prevalence ~30%) can predict prognosis Echo: concentric LVH CMR: may help identify aortic coarctation Genetics: not useful as polygenic influences Laboratory: to exclude secondary causes Others:24 h ambulatory monitoring
	Aortic stenosis	Slow rising pulse Ejection systolic murmur Soft second heart sound	ECG: LVH Echo: the trans-aortic valve gradient and the reduced valve area(beware sub-aortic membrane) CMR: nil specific Genetics: nil specific Laboratory: nil specific
	Obesity	Body mass index Waist circumference LVH regression with weight loss	ECG: attenuated LVH due to body habitus (prevalence _10%) Echo: concentric LVH, epicardial fat can predict prognosis CMR: useful if poor echo windows Genetics: monogenic disorders of body fat, e.g., leptin deficiency Laboratory: endocrine causes, e.g., diabetes, thyroid, pituitary, adrenal
Physiological LVH	Athletic heart	High level endurance training Resting bradycardia LVH regression with deconditioning	ECG: LVH Echo: mild concentric LVH (rarely>13mm) and volume loaded (dilated) LV cavity. Preserved diastolic and long axis function CMR: no late gadolinium enhancement Genetics: nil specific Laboratory: nil specific Others: VO2 max> predicted

	Condition	Clinical Pearls	Diagnostic Pointers
Sarcomere protein disease	Hypertrophic cardiomyopathy	Family history (population prevalence 1:500) Leading cause of sudden death in young athletes Risk stratification for sudden cardiac death	ECG: LVH with anterior T wave inversion, consider apical LVH. Normal PR interval. Echo: asymmetrical septal hypertrophy common (but can also present with concentric or apical LVH, and right ventricular involvement)> Normal LV dimensions in early stages of disease. Systolic anterior motion of mitral valve dilated left atrium, diastolic dysfunction, and dynamic LV outflow tract obstruction. CMR: intra-myocardial late gadolinium enhancements Genetics: autosomal dominant Laboratory: nil specific Others: end myocardial biopsy shows a triad of myocyte and myofibril disarray, myocardial fibrosis, and small vessel disease
Myocardial infiltration	Amyloidosis	Senile amyloid relatively common (20% of over 80 year olds) Multi-system involvement with variable signs including: proteinuria, peripheral, and autonomic neuropathy, hepato-splenomegaly, macroglossia	ECG: paradoxical low voltage QRS complexes, heart block, atrial fibrillation Echo: LVH with preserved LV size and biatrial dilatation, granular LV appearance (low sensitivity). Restrictive physiology and thickened inter-atrial septum and valve leaflets. CMR: global sub-endocardial late gadolinium enhancement Genetics: transthyretin gene testing (autosomal dominant) Laboratory: cross specialty investigations to differentiate between various forms of amyloid Other: Congo red staining of target organ biopsies
	Haemo-chromatosis	Late presentation in females Transfusion overload Clinical constellation includes bronze skin, arthritis, diabetes (and other endocrine abnormalities), and liver cirrhosis.	ECG: LVH Echo: LVH with biventricular and bi-atrial dilatation, restrictive physiology CMR: rapid signal decay (<20ms) on T2 imaging may guide venesection and /or iron chelation therapy Genetics: HFE gene testing (autosomal recessive) Laboratory: total body iron studies and additional investigations to evaluate complications from multi-organ iron deposition

Table 1. (Continued)

	Condition	Clinical Pearls	Diagnostic Pointers
Unclassified cardiomyopathies	Left ventricular non compaction	Familial in up to 25% of cases Also observed in other cardiomyopathies Typical presentation with triad of palpitations, thrombo-embolism, and/or heart failure	ECG:LVH, supra-ventricular arrhythmias Echo: by definition, ratio of non-compacted to compacted myocardium >2:1. Colour flow Doppler demonstration of deep perfused inter trabecular sinuses CMR: tendency to over diagnose condition Genetic: autosomal dominant in familial cases Laboratory: nil specific
Metabolic disorders	Fabry's disease	Lysosomal storage disease α-Galactosidase A deficiency Multi-system disease Enzyme replacement therapy available	ECG: LVH, short PR interval (early stages), heart block (later stages) Echo: predominant concentric LVH, right ventricular and papillary muscle hypertrophy also common CMR: late gadolinium enhancement in inferior LV wall Genetics: absence of male-male transmission due to X-linked inheritance Laboratory: proteinuria
	Pompe disease	Glycogen storage disease (type II) Acid maltase deficiency Early onset: survival beyond 1 year uncommon Late onset: can present in adulthood Limb-girdle and respiratory muscle weakness Enzyme replacement therapy available	ECG: LVH, short PR interval (early stages), accessory pathways Echo: concentric LVH with restrictive physiology CMR: nil specific Genetics: autosomal recessive Laboratory: serum CK elevated, no fasting hypoglycaemia Others: muscle biopsy
	Danon disease	Lysosomal glycogen storage disease with normal acid maltase Lysosomal-associated membrane protein 2 (LAMP2) transported protein deficiency Males present in childhood, females present in early adulthood Skeletal muscle weakness and mental retardation	ECG: LVH, short PR interval (early stages), accessory pathways Echo: concentric LVH with restrictive physiology CMR: nil specific Genetics: autosomal recessive Laboratory: normal acid maltase activity with reduced LAMP2 activity Others: muscle biopsy

	Condition	Clinical Pearls	Diagnostic Pointers
	PRKAG2 cardiomyopathy	Lysosomal glycogen storage disease AMP-activated protein kinase 2 gene mutation Multi-system involvement rare	ECG: LVH, short PR interval (early stages), accessory pathways Echo: concentric LVH with restrictive physiology CMR: nil specific Genetics: autosomal dominant
	Primary carnitine deficiency	Fatty acid oxidation disorder Functional carnitine transported deficiency Typically childhood presentation, but can present in adulthood Skeletal muscle weakness, hepatomegaly, abnormal (fatty acid metabolism)	ECG: LVH, short PR interval (early stages), accessory pathways Echo: concentric LVH with restrictive physiology CMR: nil specific Genetics: autosomal recessive Laboratory: hypoglycaemia, hyperammonaemia
Mitochondrial myopathies	Multiple varieties, e.g., Kearns-Sayre syndrome, MERFF syndrome, MELAS syndrome	Characterised by skeletal weakness and mitochondrial disease Cardiac: arrhythmias and LVH Neurology: ataxia, stroke, nystagmus, ptosis, ophthalmoplegia, retinitis pigmentosa	ECG: LVH, short PR interval (early stages), accessory pathways Echo: concentric LVH with restrictive physiology CMR: nil specific Genetics: mitochondrial DNA mutation analysis Laboratory: serum CK and glucose normal or elevated Other: muscle biopsy shows typical ragged red fibres
Syndromic conditions	Multiple varieties, examples include: Noonan syndrome: common (up to 1:1000 live births). Sporadic or autosomal dominant inheritance with mutations involving growth hormone proteins. Typically, facial dysmorphia, short stature, and cardiac abnormalities including LVH, pulmonary stenosis, septal defects Friedreich's ataxia: uncommon (up to 1:35000 live births). Autosomal recessive with mutations involving proteins associated with mitochondrial iron metabolism. Typically limb and gait ataxias, dysarthria, diabetes, and variable upper and lower motor neurone neuropathies of the lower limbs. Wheelchair bound in early adulthood. LVH presents in most cases.		

Adapted from EHJ (2013) 34, 802-808.

References

[1] Levy, D., et al., Prognostic implications of echocardiographically determined left ventricular mass in the Framingham Heart Study. *The New England journal of medicine,* 1990. 322(22): p. 1561-6.

[2] Lang, R. M., et al., Recommendations for chamber quantification: a report from the American Society of Echocardiography's Guidelines and Standards Committee and the Chamber Quantification Writing Group, developed in conjunction with the European Association of Echocardiography, a branch of the European Society of Cardiology. *Journal of the American Society of Echocardiography : official publication of the American Society of Echocardiography,* 2005. 18(12): p. 1440-63.

[3] Bos, J. M., J. A. Towbin, and M. J. Ackerman, Diagnostic, prognostic, and therapeutic implications of genetic testing for hypertrophic cardiomyopathy. *Journal of the American College of Cardiology,* 2009. 54(3): p. 201-11.

[4] Mancia, G., et al., 2013 ESH/ESC guidelines for the management of arterial hypertension: the Task Force for the Management of Arterial Hypertension of the European Society of Hypertension (ESH) and of the European Society of Cardiology (ESC). *European heart journal,* 2013. 34(28): p. 2159-219.

[5] Vahanian, A., et al., Guidelines on the management of valvular heart disease (version 2012). *European heart journal,* 2012. 33(19): p. 2451-96.

[6] PH53, N.g., Managing overweight and obesity in adults – lifestyle weight management services. 2014.

[7] Maron, B. J., et al., American College of Cardiology/European Society of Cardiology Clinical Expert Consensus Document on Hypertrophic Cardiomyopathy. A report of the American College of Cardiology Foundation Task Force on Clinical Expert Consensus Documents and the European Society of Cardiology Committee for Practice Guidelines. *European heart journal,* 2003. 24(21): p. 1965-91.

[8] Falk, R. H., Diagnosis and management of the cardiac amyloidoses. *Circulation,* 2005. 112(13): p. 2047-60.

[9] Bacon, B. R., et al., Diagnosis and management of hemochromatosis: 2011 practice guideline by the American Association for the Study of Liver Diseases. *Hepatology,* 2011. 54(1): p. 328-43.

[10] Schaefer, R. M., A. Tylki-Szymanska, and M. J. Hilz, Enzyme replacement therapy for Fabry disease: a systematic review of available evidence. *Drugs,* 2009. 69(16): p. 2179-205.

[11] Weidemann, F., et al., Long-term effects of enzyme replacement therapy on fabry cardiomyopathy: evidence for a better outcome with early treatment. *Circulation,* 2009. 119(4): p. 524-9.

[12] Weidemann, F., et al., Cardiac challenges in patients with Fabry disease. *International journal of cardiology,* 2010. 141(1): p. 3-10.

In: Left Ventricular Hypertrophy (LVH)
Editor: Richard T. Matthews

ISBN: 978-1-63463-022-1
© 2015 Nova Science Publishers, Inc.

Chapter 5

Preclinical Carotid Pathology and Cardiac Remodeling in Hypertension in Aging

M. Otero-Losada, Sc.D., Ph.D.[1]; D. Sanchez Gelós, M.D.[1];
F. Azzato, M.D., Ph.D.[1]; H. Gómez Llambí, M.D.[1];
G. Ambrosio, M.D., Ph.D.[2] and J. Milei, M.D., Ph.D.[1]

[1] Instituto de Investigaciones Cardiológicas, ININCA.UBA.CONICET, Buenos Aires, Argentina
[2] Cardiologia e Fisiopatologia Cardiovascolare, Università di Perugia, Italy

Abstract

The aim of this study is to assess whether carotid lesion might reflect preclinical target organ damage (TOD) and its relationship with cardiac remodeling in hypertension in aging. Patients (n=93) underwent electro- and echocardiographic evaluation, 24-hr Holter recording, BP monitoring, pulse wave velocity (PWV) determinations and routine analyses. Carotid damage was associated with an increase in diurnal and nocturnal systolic BP variability (BPVar) even after controlling for age, sex and body mass index. Eccentric remodeling was related to diastolic BPVar (p<0.05), diurnal systolic BPVar (p <0.02) and plaque atheroma development (p<0.001). Concentric remodeling was related to PWV variation (p<0.03). Patients with left ventricle hypertrophy showed higher prevalence of carotid atheroma (62% vs 33% normal geometry, p<0.01). The relationship between carotid damage and increased BPVar suggests a role for the former as a sign of preclinical TOD. Cardiac geometry might prove a reliable indicator of cardiovascular risk in hypertension in aging.

Keywords: Hypertension; carotid damage; cardiac remodeling; left ventricle hypertrophy; blood pressure variability

Introduction

Alteration in circadian blood pressure and high blood pressure variability (BPVar) may cause left ventricular hypertrophy (LVH) [1-4], a well-recognized risk factor for cardiovascular events [5] whereas arterial stiffness alters baroreceptor sensitivity, which in turn affects BPVar perpetuating a vicious cycle [6]. In this respect, we recently described a relationship between morning surge in blood pressure (MS), autonomic dysfunction, and target organ damage (TOD) at the vascular level (increased arterial stiffness) and in the heart (increased left ventricular mass) in older subjects [6].

The search for accurate, simple, and reliable indicators of preclinical TOD remains an issue of utmost importance in the management of patients with hypertension. Even though issues related to carotid wall injury have been explored in hypertensive [7] and healthy men [8], the complex interplay between carotid damage (extra-cardiac TOD), BPVar, arterial stiffness and cardiac remodeling (cardiac damage) have rarely been evaluated.

Carotid intima–media thickness is a powerful and independent indicator of arteriosclerosis, pointing out to an early involvement of target organ in essential hypertension [9]. Recently, increasing age and LVH were associated with high prevalence of both left ventricle concentric remodeling and carotid wall damage [10]. Yet, limited information is available on the relationship between early extra-cardiac organ damage and remodeling patterns of the left ventricle in hypertension, particularly in the elderly.

Accordingly, the present study was carried out in order to get insights into carotid wall damage as a sign of preclinical TOD and its relationship with cardiac geometry in hypertension in aging. To this goal, arterial stiffness and cardiac geometry were evaluated in elderly hypertensive subjects undergoing clinical and echocardiographic evaluation, 24-hr arterial blood pressure monitoring (ABPM) and pulse wave velocity (PWV) determinations.

Materials and Methods

Ninety-three consecutive outpatients were enrolled in this study. Twenty-four men and 69 women (76±2 and 74±1 years old, respectively; age range 65-91 years) were clinically and neurologically assessed. Inclusion criteria: hypertensive subjects over 65 years old under treatment and controlled (i.e., subjects were normotensive at the time of the study). Exclusion criteria: bradycardia, treatment with beta-blockers, arrhythmias (including atrial fibrillation), severe anemia, diabetic autonomic neuropathy, Guillain-Barré syndrome and heart failure [11, 2].

Hypertensive patients treated with angiotensin-converting enzyme inhibitors, diuretics, and/or calcium antagonists continued treatments after inclusion in the protocol. Routine laboratory and electrocardiographic evaluations were performed. Blood pressure was measured after a 5-min rest period in the sitting position at the clinical office using an automatic blood pressure monitor (Omron Hem-742INT, Omron Healthcare, INC, Norway). Noninvasive ABPM was performed for 24 hours using automatic devices (ABPM-Spacelab 90207-30, SpaceLab Inc. Redmond, Washington; USA) which recorded blood pressure and heart rate every 15 minutes during day time and every 20 minutes in the night. Sleep-through

MS was defined as the mean systolic blood pressure (SBP) during the 2 hours after awakening minus the mean SBP of the hour that included the lowest sleep SBP [2].

Ambulatory blood pressure variability was estimated as the standard deviation of the 24-hr mean (systolic and diastolic) blood pressure recording [3]. Pulse wave velocity (PWV) was measured along the descending thoracoabdominal aorta using the validated foot-to-foot velocity method [3]. Briefly, waveforms were obtained transcutaneously over the common carotid artery and the right femoral artery, and the time delay (t) was measured between the feet of the two waveforms. The distance (D) covered by the waves was assimilated to the distance measured between the two recording sites. Pulse wave velocity was calculated as PWV=D/t (meters/second) [12].

Carotid artery evaluation was performed with patients lying in the dorsal decubitus position, with the head slightly turned toward the opposite side of the carotid artery under examination. An ATL Apogee CX echocardiographic machine equipped with a 7.5-MHz transducer was used. A 3.5-MHz transducer was used in case of high carotid bifurcations in order to examine the full stretch of the internal carotid artery [13].

This investigation was conducted with the approval of the Bioethics Committee of the Instituto de Investigaciones Cardiológicas "Profesor Dr. Alberto C. Taquini", Facultad de Medicina, University of Buenos Aires with respect to clinical care and laboratory investigation and in conformity to the ethical guidelines of the 1975 Declaration of Helsinki.

Statistical Procedures

After a multiple analysis of variance (MANOVA), data were submitted to multidimensional scaling and bivariate correlation analyses (Pearson's product moment correlation coefficient) to evaluate the degree of association between pairs of variables.To evaluate whether specific factors of interest were involved in the associations or just spurious variation (confounders), one-way ANOVA followed by a post-hoc test (LSD, Bonferroni) was used when appropiate.The level of statistical significance was set at p<0.05. Data plotting and analyses were performed using the SPSS™ statistical package version 17.0 (SPSS Inc., Chicago, USA).

Results

Table 1 shows the clinical and demographic characteristics of study population. All patients had normal office BP values at the time of the study. Overall prevalence of LVH (left ventricular mass >117 g/m^2 in men and >104 g/m^2 in women) was 52%; carotid thickened wall and/or non-obstructing plaque atheroma were found in 23% of subjects.

Carotid involvement was associated with increased 24-hr SBPVar (38% explained variance, p<0.01). The coexistence of carotid wall pathology and increased blood pressure or dipping behavior was associated with the largest increases in the 24-hr SBPVar. However, neither increased blood pressure nor dipping behaviors were independently related to changes in SBPVar (Figure 1). Actually, carotid wall damage was associated with SBPVar throughout the 24 hr cycle regardless of whether diurnal (r=0.311, p<0.03), nocturnal (r=0.340, p<0.02), or daily (24hr) (r=0.363, p<0.01) values were analyzed even after controlling for age, sex and body mass index (Figure 2). Accordingly, MS was related to SBPVar, DBPVar and mean BPVar regardless of whether diurnal, nocturnal or daily fluctuation was evaluated (p<0.0001).

Table 1. Clinical and demographic characteristics of the study population

Group	Subgroup	n	% within group
Fasting glycemia	Normal	78	84
	High	15	16
Sedentarism	No	76	82
	Yes	17	18
Dislipemia	No	55	59
	Yes	38	41
Smoking	No	64	68
	Yes	29	32
Carotid wall	Normal	39	42
	Damaged (*)	54	58
Plaque atheroma (non obstructive)	No	55	60
	Yes	38	40
Dipping condition	Dipper	54	58
	Non dipper	39	42
Sex	Female	68	73
	Male	25	27

(*) carotid thickening with or without non obstructive plaque.

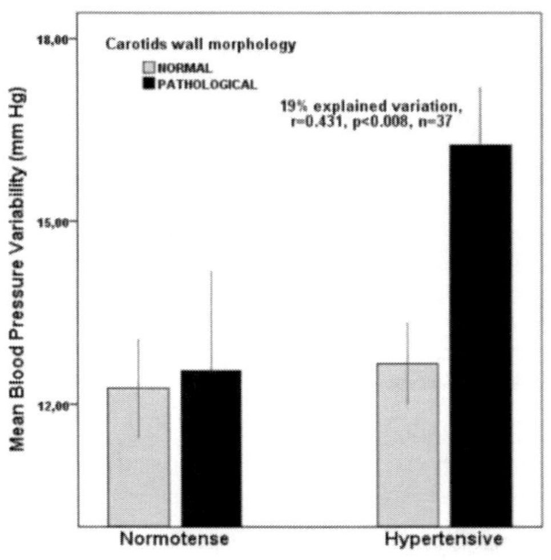

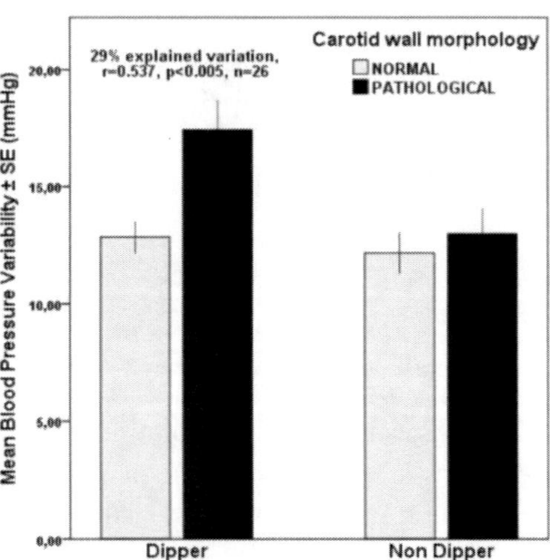

*p< 0.01 vs corresponding normal carotids.

Figure 1. Relationship between the 24-hr systolic blood pressure variability and carotid wall damage: dependence on hypertension (left) and dipping condition (right).

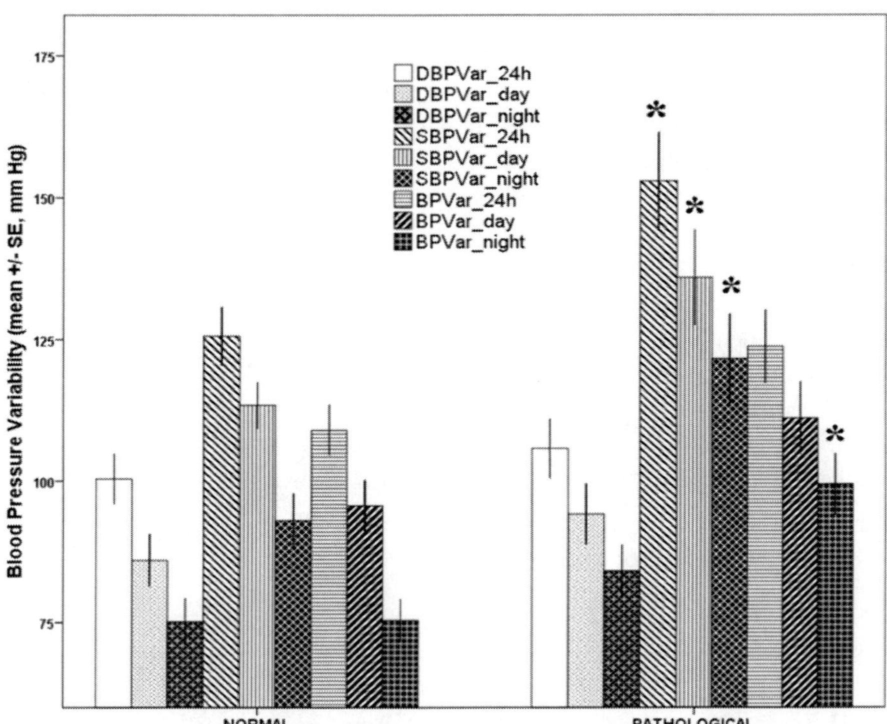

*p<0.03 (diurnal), *p<0.02 (nocturnal), *p<0.01 (24hr) vs. normal carotids for SBPVar:
*p<0.03 vs normal carotid for 24hr-MBPVar.

Figure 2. Relationship between carotid wall damage and blood pressure variability.

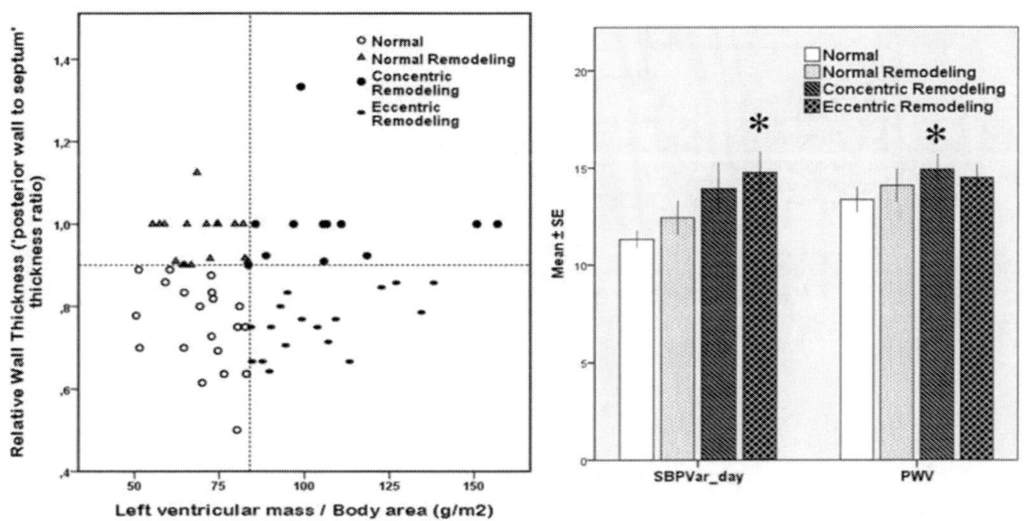

*p <0.02 vs normal heart for diurnal SBPVar; *p<0.03 vs normal heart, vs normal remodeling, vs
   eccentric remodeling for PWV.

Figure 3. Cardiac geometry: relative wall thickness and left ventricular mass values in the study
population (left). 24-hr systolic blood pressure variability and pulse wave velocity values according
with left ventricular remodeling pattern (right).

Cardiac geometry data are depicted in Figure 3. Overall correlation was found for heart remodeling with DBPVar (r=-0.228, p<0.04), diurnal SBPVar (r=0.318, p<0.01), and presence of carotid plaque atheroma (r=0.465, p<0.001). Eccentric remodeling was associated with DBPVar (p<0.05), diurnal SBPVar (p <0.02), and presence of plaque atheroma (p<0.001), compared with normal hearts (Figure 3 left). In contrast, concentric remodeling was associated with changes in PWV compared with any other remodeling pattern (p<0.03) (Figure 3 right). Removal of potentially confounding factors from the model (simultaneously controlling for the effects of age, sex, BMI, dislipemia, fasting hyperglycemia) had no appreciable effect on the above correlations in all cases, indicating that those factors were not related to cardiac geometry.

Prevalence of carotid pathology was higher in patients with LVH compared with those showing normal ventricular size: 62% vs 33% (p<0.01).

Left atrium enlargement was found more often in patients with concentric LV remodeling compared with those with normal heart (p<0.003) and normal remodeling (p<0.006).

Figure 4 schematically shows the associations among some of the cardiovascular parameters explored in this paper.

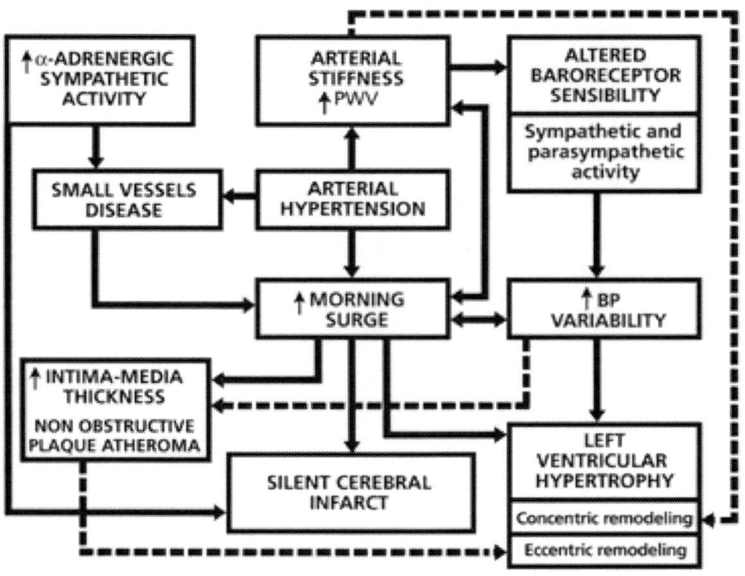

Figure 4.

Discussion

In this paper, carotid wall abnormalities were associated with an increase in SBPVar throughout the 24 hr cycle, regardless of diurnal, nocturnal or daily fluctuation, or whether carotid thickening or plaque were considered. Recently, we reported the association between MS and the 24-hr SBPVar in the same patients [6]. Further analysis revealed a wider linkage between MS and BP variability regardless of the measure considered (SBPVar, DBPVar and mean BPVar either diurnal, nocturnal or daily). Lately, Verdecchia et al. shed light on the prognostic value of early MS in 3012 untreated subjects with essential hypertension [4]. There was a direct association between BP dip from day to night and the BP surge after awakening and an unexpected increase in the risk of cardiovascular events in patients with blunted MS. The authors suggested the use of 24-hour SBP and a blunted or reversed fall in SBP from day to night as independent variables for cardiovascular risk stratification. Association between awake SBPVar and TOD has been reported in long standing hypertension [14, 15] and in newly diagnosed hypertension [16]. In this connection, Verdecchia et al., [14] examined data of 2545 untreated hypertensive subjects and demonstrated that the association between pulse pressure and left ventricular mass is explained by SBP, which is the main pressure determinant of left ventricular mass in essential hypertension.

The overall prevalence of LVH (52%) and carotid damage (23%) in our study is in agreement with a previous report (51% and 24% respectively) [17].

We also observed that the prevalence of carotid plaque pathology was higher in patients with LVH compared with those showing normal ventricular size. Interestingly, not long ago, the same observation was reported in aging untreated hypertensives, but not in young hypertensives [10]. If these findings were confirmed in future studies, the relationship between plaque atheroma and cardiac remodeling may not benefit from antihypertensive treatment in the elderly.

Combining relative wall thickness (RWT) with the value of LV mass allowed to identify subgroups of patients according with LV hypertrophy (LVH) and the type of geometric remodeling [18]. Eccentric remodeling was associated with diurnal SBP values and existence of carotid plaque atheroma, while concentric remodeling was related to arterial stiffness (PWV). Our findings are supported by a previous report about the impact of arterial stiffening on left ventricular structure [19]. However remodeling patterns were not related to BP differences. Eccentric remodeling was associated with carotid wall pathology (arterial TOD) while concentric remodeling was related to hardening of the vessels. Present correlation between cardiac geometry, mean BP and DBP are in agreement with the classical belief [20]. Nevertheless, factors other than BP might contribute to the phenotypical expression of cardiac remodeling at least in treated hypertension in aging [21].

Classically, left ventricular concentric remodeling was considered as an adaptive change in cardiac geometry frequently observed in arterial hypertension [22]. Cuspidi et al. investigated the extent of TOD in patients with left ventricular concentric remodeling and concluded that in hypertensive patients with similar BP and left ventricular mass index, concentric remodeling was not associated with more prominent extra-cardiac TOD [22]. Consistent with ours, their findings show that geometric patterns are concomitant with subclinical extra-cardiac alterations and may be regarded as a reliable marker of cardiovascular risk [23].

The present relationship between PWV and concentric remodeling has been reported in aged but not in young people [24]. The finding that left atrium enlargement was observed in patients with concentric remodeling is supported by an earlier study [22].

In agreement with our previous report, MS was closely correlated to PWV and 24-hr SBPVar in all patients [2]. High BPVar and MS are known to be associated with LVH, whereas arterial stiffness alters barorreceptor sensitivity, in turn affecting BPVar and perpetuating a vicious cycle.

Speculation made on how this is a self-perpetuating cycle (drawn from Figure 4) is intended to outline what is usually observed in the clinical practice. Nevertheless, understanding cardiac remodeling in essential hypertension in aging has still a way to go.

The small number of subjects in this study limits the extrapolation of present findings; also, our data do not allow to speculate about possible events at follow up.

Conclusion

Cardiac remodeling was related to changes in DBPVar and diurnal SBPVar. Carotid damage was associated with increased SBPVar and heart remodeling pattern. Carotid injury might be an important marker of extra-cardiac end-organ damage in elderly patients with essential hypertension.

Acknowledgments

The authors thank Mariana Milei for her expert collaboration with graphical design.

Funding. This study received financial support from National Research Council CONICET [PIP 6549] and the University of Buenos Aires, Argentina [UBACYT M052].

Declaration of Conflicting Interests. The authors declare that they have no conflicts of interest competing financial interests, relationships and affiliations relevant to the subject of this manuscript.

The experiments reported in this paper were performed under a Framework Agreement between the University of Buenos Aires (Buenos Aires, Argentina) and the University of Perugia, School of Medicine (Perugia, Italy).

References

[1]   Fagard RH, Thijs L, Staessen JA, Clement DL, De Buyzere ML, De Bacquer DA. Night-day blood pressure ratio and dipping pattern as predictors of death and cardiovascular events in hypertension. *J Hum Hypertens* 2009; 23: 645-53

[2]   Kario K. Vascular damage in exaggerated morning surge in blood pressure. *Hypertension* 2007; 49: 771-772

[3]   Parati G, Pomidossi G, Albini F, Malaspina D, Mancia G. Relationship of 24-hour blood pressure means and variability to severity of target organ damage in hypertension. *J Hypertens* 1987; 5: 93-98

[4]   Verdecchia P, Angeli F, Mazzotta G, Garofoli M, Ramundo E, Gentile G, Ambrosio G, Reboldi G. Day-night dip and early-morning surge in blood pressure in hypertension: prognostic implications. *Hypertension* 2012; 60: 34-42

[5]   Verdecchia P, Porcellati C, Reboldi G, Gattobigio R, Borgioni C, Pearson TA, Ambrosio G. Left ventricular hypertrophy as an independent predictor of acute cerebrovascular events in essential hypertension. *Circulation* 2001; 104: 2039-44

[6]   Sanchez Gelós DF, Otero-Losada ME, Azzato F, Milei J. Morning surge, pulse wave velocity, and autonomic function tests in elderly adults. *Blood Press Monit* 2012; 17: 103-109

[7]   Bigazzi R, Bianchi S, Nenci R, Baldari D, Baldari G, Campese VM. Increased thickness of the carotid artery in patients with essential hypertension and microalbuminuria. *J Hum Hypertens* 1995; 9: 827-833

[8]   Agewall S, Bjorn F. Microalbuminuria and intima media thickness of the carotid artery in clinically healthy men. *Atherosclerosis* 2002; 164: 161-166

[9]   Takiuchi S, Kamide K, Miwa Y, Tomiyama M, Yoshii M, Matayoshi T et al. Diagnostic value of carotid intima-media thickness and plaque score for predicting target organ damage in patients with essential hypertension. *J Hum Hypertens* 2004; 18: 17–23

[10]   Cuspidi C, Meani S, Sala C, Valerio C, Negri F, Mancia G. Age related prevalence of severe left ventricular hypertrophy in essential hypertension: echocardiographic findings from the ETODH study. *Blood Press* 2012: 139-45

[11]   Milei J, Lavezzi AM, Bruni B, Grana DR, Azzato F, Matturri L. Carotid barochemoreceptor pathological findings regarding carotid plaque status and aging. *Can J Cardiol* 2009; 25: e6-e12

[12]   Laurent S, Boutouyrie P, Asmar R, Gautier I, Laloux B, Guize L, et al. Aortic stiffness is an independent predictor of all-cause and cardiovascular mortality in hypertensive patients. *Hypertension* 2001; 37: 1236-41

[13]   Beigelman R, Izaguirre A, Robles M, Grana D, Ambrosio G, Milei J. Kinking of carotid arteries is not a mechanism of cerebral ischemia: a functional evaluation by Doppler echography. *Int Angiol* 2011; 30: 342-8

[14]   Verdecchia P, Schillaci G, Borgioni C, Gattobigio R, Ambrosio G, Porcellati C. Prevalent influence of systolic over pulse pressure on left ventricular mass in essential hypertension. *Eur Heart J.* 2002; 23: 658-65

[15]   Tatasciore A, Renda G, Zimarino M, Soccio M, Bilo G, Parati G et al. Awake systolic blood pressure variability correlates with target-organ damage in hypertensive subjects. *Hypertension* 2007; 50:325-32

[16]   Tatasciore A, Zimarino M, Renda G, Zurro M, Soccio M, Prontera C et al. Awake blood pressure variability, inflammatory markers and target organ damage in newly diagnosed hypertension. *Hypertens Res* 2008; 31:2137-46

[17]   Leoncini G, Sacchi G, Ravera M, Viazzi F, Ratto E, Vettoretti S, Parodi D, Bezante GP, Del Sette M, Deferrari G, Pontremoli R. Microalbuminuria is an integrated marker of subclinical organ damage in primary hypertension. *J Hum Hypertens* 2002; 16: 399-404

[18]   Ganau A, Devereux RB, Roman MJ, de Simone G, Pickering TG, Saba PS, Vargiu P, Simongini I, Laragh JH. Patterns of left ventricular hypertrophy and geometric remodeling in essential hypertension. *J Am Coll Cardiol* 1992; 19: 1550-8

[19]   Roman MJ, Ganau A, Saba PS, Pini R, Pickering TG, Devereux RB. Impact of arterial stiffening on left ventricular structure. *Hypertension* 2000; 36:489-94

[20]   Devereux RB, Roman MJ. Left ventricular hypertrophy in hypertension: stimuli, patterns, and consequences. *Hypertens Res* 1999; 22:1-9

[21] de Simone G, Daniels SR, Kimball TR, Roman MJ, Romano C, Chinali M et al. Evaluation of concentric left ventricular geometry in humans: evidence for age-related systematic underestimation. *Hypertension* 2005; 45:64-8

[22] Cuspidi C, Macca G, Michev I, Fusi V, Severgnini B, Corti C et al. Left ventricular concentric remodeling and extracardiac target organ damage in essential hypertension. *J Hum Hypertens* 2002; 16: 385-90

[23] Cuspidi C, Giudici V, Negri F, Sala C, Mancia G. Left ventricular geometry, ambulatory blood pressure and extra-cardiac organ damage in untreated essential hypertension. *Blood Press Monit* 2010; 15: 124-31

[24] Schillaci G, Mannarino MR, Pucci G, Pirro M, Helou J, Savarese G, Vaudo G, Mannarino E. Age-specific relationship of aortic pulse wave velocity with left ventricular geometry and function in hypertension. *Hypertension* 2007; 49:317-2

In: Left Ventricular Hypertrophy (LVH) ISBN: 978-1-63463-022-1
Editor: Richard T. Matthews © 2015 Nova Science Publishers, Inc.

Chapter 6

Predictive Factors Associated with Left Ventricular Hypertrophy in Pre-Dialysis and Dialysis Patients

Hiroaki Io and Yasuhiko Tomino[*]
Division of Nephrology, Department of Internal Medicine,
Juntendo University Faculty of Medicine, Tokyo, Japan

Abstract

Background: Currently, left ventricular (LV) hypertrophy and dysfunction are considered to be the strongest predictors of cardiovascular mortality in chronic kidney disease (CKD) patients. We investigated the factors associated with elevated LV mass index (LVMI) using echocardiography and assessed the therapeutic implications of strategies used to treat CKD (stages 1–5D) patients.

Methods: We prospectively determined correlations among biochemical values, physical specimens, and LVMI using echocardiography in 30 nondiabetic hemodialysis (HD) and 32 peritoneal dialysis (PD) (stage 5D) patients. These parameters were measured at 0 (baseline), 12, and 24 months after initiation of dialysis. Physical, biochemical, and LVMI data evaluated using echocardiography were also retrospectively analyzed in 930 CKD (stages 1–5) patients.

Results: In HD patients, LVMI values at 12 and 24 months were not significantly decreased compared with those at baseline. Systolic blood pressure (SBP), residual glomerular filtration rate, and serum albumin levels at baseline were identified as independent risk factors for LVMI in multivariate regression analysis. In PD patients, LVMI values at 12 and 24 months were significantly decreased compared with those at baseline ($p < 0.05$). Plasma atrial natriuretic peptide (ANP) was significantly correlated with left atrium diameter (LAD) and LVMI. In CKD (stages 4–5) patients, SBP, serum albumin levels, and left atrium volume index measured using echocardiography were identified as independent risk factors for duration before initiation of dialysis on

---

[*] Address correspondence and reprint requests to: Yasuhiko Tomino M.D., Division of Nephrology, Department of Internal Medicine, Juntendo University Faculty of Medicine, 2-1-1 Hongo, Bunkyo-ku, Tokyo 113-8421, Japan, Tel and Fax: +81-3-5802-1064 or -1065, E-mail: yasu@juntendo.ac.jp.

multivariate regression analysis. In CKD (stage 1–5) patients, LVMI increased with decreasing renal function. Levels of SBP and hemoglobin (Hb) were independent risk factors for LVMI in the multivariate regression analysis. In the patients who showed worsening LVMI, the rates of change in SBP, proteinuria, and Hb were identified as independent risk factors for LVMI changes.

Conclusions: It is difficult to improve LVH in HD patients. Plasma ANP and LAD measurements showed that left ventricular structure, contraction, and compliance were well preserved in PD patients undergoing aggressive treatment. It is important to treat hypertension and overhydration on the basis of plasma ANP and Hb levels before initiating dialysis. Our findings may have some therapeutic implications for the strategies used to treat predialysis and dialysis patients.

Keywords: CKD, LVMI, dialysis, LVH, hypertension, anemia

Introduction

The incidence of end-stage kidney disease (ESKD) is steadily increasing around the world. Cardiovascular disease (CVD) is the main cause of morbidity and mortality in pre-dialysis CKD patients [1] [2]. Deaths associated with CVD in dialysis patients are 10–30 times more frequent than those in the general population. CVD is also responsible for up to 50% of the all-cause mortality rate [5]. Cardiovascular involvement in CKD patients primarily manifests as left ventricular (LV) hypertrophy (LVH) and LV dysfunction [3] [4]. LVH is recognized as a potent risk factor for cardiovascular death in dialysis patients [6]; it is a strong predictor of myocardial infarction, cardiac failure, sudden death, and stroke [7]. Regression of LVH lowers the incidence of major cardiovascular events and improves survival rate [8]. The left atrium (LA) diameter defined by echocardiography has been reported to be directly related to the risk of cardiovascular death, and the association of LA enlargement with cardiovascular death appears to be partially related to LVH [9]. Currently, LVH and LV dysfunction are considered to be the strongest predictors of cardiovascular mortality in dialysis patients. The synthesis of cardiac natriuretic peptides was increased with alterations in LV mass and function. We aimed to investigate the factors associated with elevated LV mass index (LVMI) using echocardiography and to discuss therapeutic implications for the strategies used to treat CKD patients.

Methods

1. Prospective Study Cohort

The prospective study cohort consisted of 30 hemodialysis (HD) (17 males, 13 females) and 32 peritoneal dialysis (PD) (24 males, 8 females) patients treated in the Juntendo University Hospital from April 2002 to April 2008. The enrollment criteria included no history of congestive heart failure (defined as dyspnea or interstitial edema on chest X-ray), valvular disease, left ventricular systolic dysfunction with an ejection fraction <50%, arrhythmia or abnormal electrocardiography. Diabetic patients were excluded from this study.

All patients had arterio-venous fistulas created before initiation of HD and before enrollment into the study.

All patients were treated with an angiotensin type 1 receptor blocker to maintain blood pressure (BP) at <140/90 mmHg. Other antihypertensive drugs, such as diuretics and/or calcium channel blockers (CCB), were added if BP increased to >140/90 mmHg. Other basic markers of volume status, such as clinical features of volume overload (edema and heart failure symptoms), were also examined. Body fluid balance was controlled by measuring plasma atrial natriuretic peptide [ANP: normal range, <43.0 pg/ml (10)] and LA diameter [LAD; normal range, <39 mm [9]]. A diuretic was given to the patients who decreased their water intake if plasma ANP was >43.0 pg/ml or LAD >39 mm.

Echocardiographic Examinations

The echocardiographic examinations were performed before or at the start of dialysis (baseline) and at 12 and 24 months. Based on the baseline LVMI, HD patients were divided into three groups: group A (normal), <125 g/m^2; group B (mild-moderate LVH), 125–175 g/m^2; and group C (moderate-severe LVH), >175 g/m^2. The protocol conformed to the ethical guidelines of our institutions, and informed consent was obtained from all participants.

2. Retrospective Study Design

The enrollment criteria were patients who had undergone routine laboratory measurements and transthoracic echocardiography between 1999 and 2009 in the Juntendo University Hospital, Tokyo, Japan. Patients underwent echocardiography in the hospital on routine visits to the outpatient clinic.

Patients on dialysis treatment with renal transplants were excluded. We enrolled 930 patients with CKD (610 males and 320 females). The study was conducted in accordance with the Declaration of Helsinki and institutional guidelines, and the protocol was approved by the Ethics Committee of Juntendo University Hospital.

Echocardiographic Examinations

A retrospective longitudinal study was performed on 109 CKD patients before starting dialysis (73 males, 36 females). The clinical, laboratory, and urine parameters were recorded at baseline and in the follow-up period (21.2 ± 17.9 months). These parameters were compared by calculating the rates of change [(baseline − follow-up)/ baseline].

Echocardiographic examinations, including cardiac hypertrophy examinations and two-dimensional and M-mode echocardiography, were performed by using a Toshiba ultrasound system (Model 260 SS-A equipped with a 2.5-MHz phased-array transducer; Toshiba Corp., Tokyo, Japan) in all patients by an experienced investigator. Echocardiographic examinations were performed on a nondialysis day. All examinations were performed with the patient in the left lateral position, and all echocardiographic data were evaluated according to the guidelines of the American Society of Echocardiography [11]. LA and ventricular size, intraventricular septal thickness, posterior left ventricular wall thickness, and the LV mass were recorded [12].

LV mass was corrected by the body surface area and expressed as LVMI [13]. The severity of LVH was assessed by LVMI. Left atrial volume index (LAVi) was calculated according to the prolate ellipse method [14].

Statistical Analyses

All data were expressed as mean ± standard deviations. Student's t-test was used to analyze the differences in the average values between the unpaired groups. Student's t-test or Fisher's exact test were used to perform univariate analysis. Stepwise linear regression analysis using a forward–backward procedure was used to analyze variables with p-values <0.05 in the univariate analysis. The F-value for entry or removal of candidate variables from the discriminant function was set at 4.0. Repeated analysis of variance was performed for comparisons of serial changes in the clinical data and echocardiographic parameters. Stat View version 5.0 (HULINKS) was used to perform all calculations. $P < 0.05$ was considered to indicate statistical significance.

Results

1. CKD (Stage 5D: HD) Patients

LVMI was 115.9 ± 12.7 g/m^2 in group A (normal), 161.2 ± 7.7 g/m^2 in group B (mild–moderate LVH), and 202.9 ± 21.3 g/m^2 in group C (moderate–severe LVH) at the initiation of HD and 133.7 ± 21.3 g/m^2 in group A, 140.9 ± 40.7 g/m^2 in group B, and 182.1 ± 55.9 g/m^2 in group C after 24 months. LVMI was not significantly changed at 12 and 24 months compared with baseline in each group (Figure 1). LVMI in all groups at initiation of HD was not significantly different at 24 months (161.8 ± 40.2 g/m^2 vs. 148.3 ± 42.5 g/m^2, respectively).

In the univariate analysis, there were significant correlations between LVMI and systolic blood pressure (SBP), diastolic blood pressure (DBP), residual glomerular filtration ratio (rGFR), and serum albumin (Alb) levels at initiation of HD. SBP, DBP, rGFR, and ALB levels were identified as independent risk factors for LVMI in the multivariate regression analysis (Table 1).

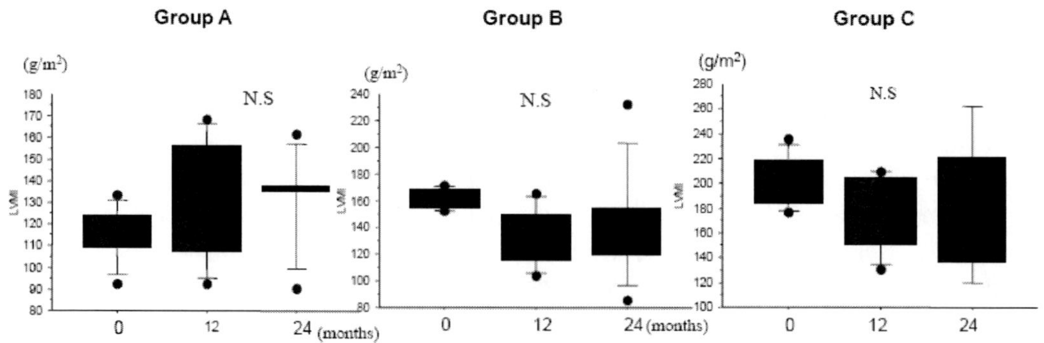

Figure 1. Follow-up of LVMI of HD patients in each group. Group A (n = 9) LVMI is <125 g/m^2, group B (n = 10) LVMI is from 125 to 175 g/m^2, and group C (n = 11) LVMI is >175 g/m^2.

Table 1. Stepwise linear regression analysis of factors associated with LVMI at initiation of HD

	P value	R value	F value
SBP	p<0.01	R=0.619	14.88
DBP	p<0.05	R=0.659	5.37
rGFR	p<0.05	R=-0.420	4.01
Alb	p<0.05	R=-0.417	4.03
Hb	p=0.250	R=-0.260	
hANP	p=0.181	R=0.330	
EPO	p=0.840	R=0.490	
Int-PTH	p=0.101	R=-0.367	

At initiation of HD

Abbreviations: EPO: Dose of erythropoietin /month, int-PTH:intact parathyroid hormone, SBP:systolic BP, DBP:diastolic BP, Alb:albumin.

2. CKD (Stage 5D: PD) Patients

LAD was 36 ± 4.6 mm at the start of dialysis and was significantly decreased to 33 ± 3.2 mm at 12 months ($p < 0.05$) and 33 ± 3.6 mm at 24 months of dialysis ($p < 0.05$). LVMI was 156 ± 45.7 g/m^2 at the start and significantly decreased to 128 ± 25.0g/m^2 at 12 months and 129 ± 30.4g/m^2 at 24 months of dialysis ($p < 0.05$) (Figure 2). ANP at the start of dialysis (56.2 ± 39.7 pg/ml) was significantly decreased to 37.7 ± 25.5 pg/ml at 12 months and 33.3 ± 19.5 pg/ml at 24 months of dialysis ($p < 0.05$) (Figure 3). ANP was significantly correlated with LAD ($R = 0.412$, $p < 0.01$), transmitral A wave flow velocity ($R = 0.429$, $p < 0.01$), and LVMI ($R = 0.426$, $p < 0.01$) (Figure 4).

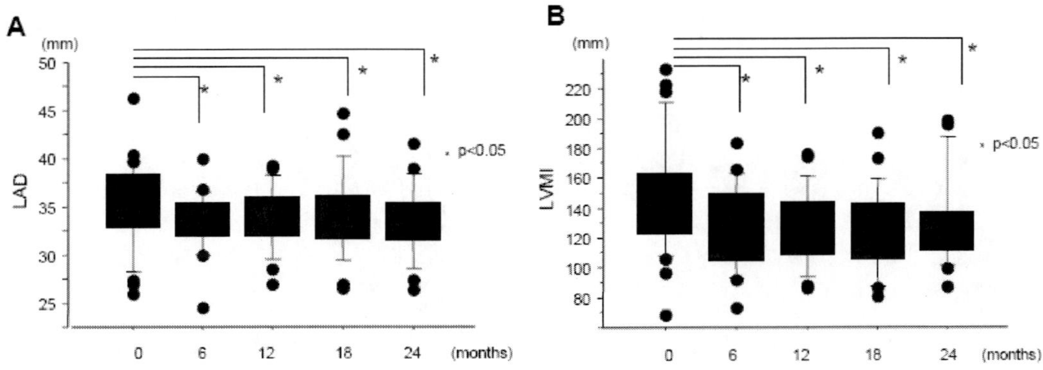

Figure 2. (Continued).

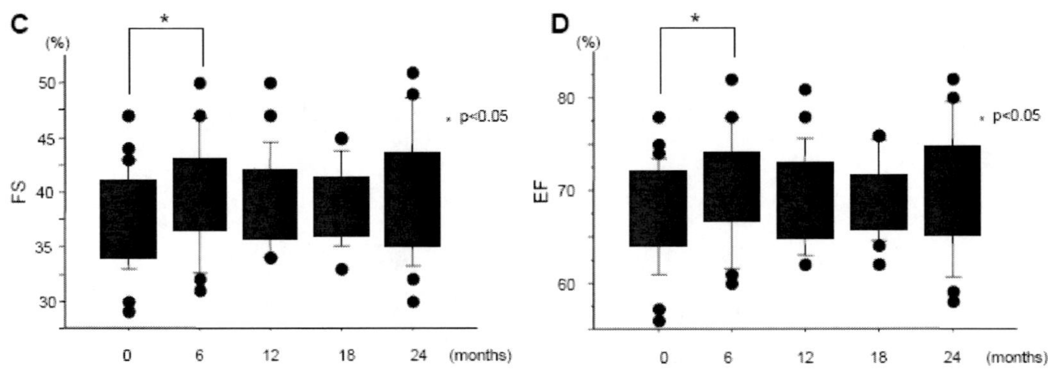

Figure 2. Follow-up echocardiographic data of PD patients. A: LAD values at 6, 12, 18, and 24 months are significantly decreased relative to those at the start of dialysis (p < 0.05). B: Left ventricular mass index (LVMI) values at 6, 12, 18, and 24 months are significantly decreased relative to those at the start of dialysis (p < 0.05). C: FS is significantly increased after 6 months relative to that at the start of dialysis (p < 0.05). D: EF is significantly increased after 6 months relative to that at the start of dialysis (p < 0.05).

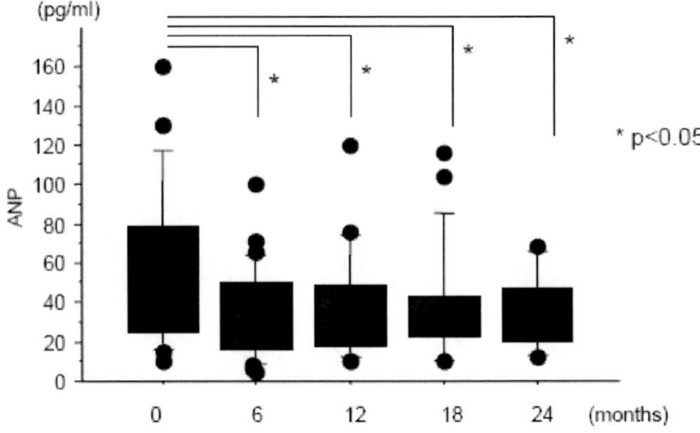

Figure 3. Follow-up plasma ANP levels of PD patients. ANP values after 6, 12, 18, and 24 months of dialysis are significantly decreased relative to those at the start of dialysis (p < 0.05).

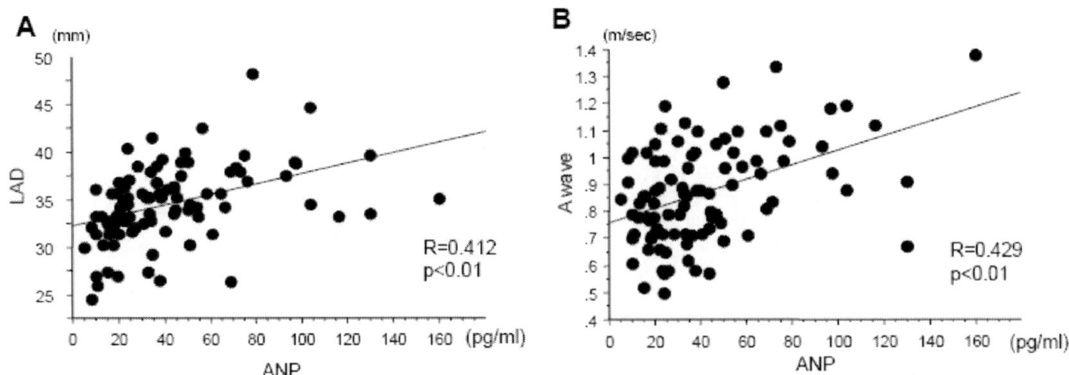

Figure 4. (Continued).

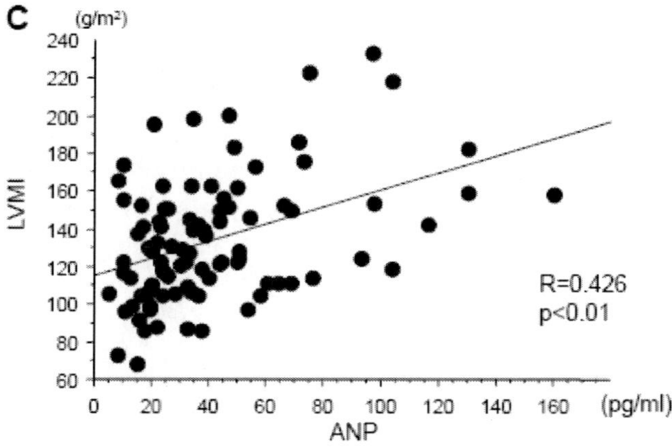

Figure 4. Correlation between plasma ANP level and echocardiographic data of PD patients. ANP is significantly correlated with A) LAD (R = 0.412, p < 0.01), B) transmitral A wave flow velocity (R = 0.429, p < 0.01), and C) LVMI (R = 0.426, p < 0.01).

3. CKD (Stage 1–5) Cross-Sectional Study

In the stepwise logistic regression analysis, levels of SBP, LAVi, and Alb were independent risk factors for duration before initiation of HD in CKD (stage 4–5). There was a significant correlation between LAVi and duration before initiation of HD (iHD). As LA volume increased, the duration before iHD decreased, which meant that the severity of diastolic dysfunction reflected the duration before iHD (Figure 5).

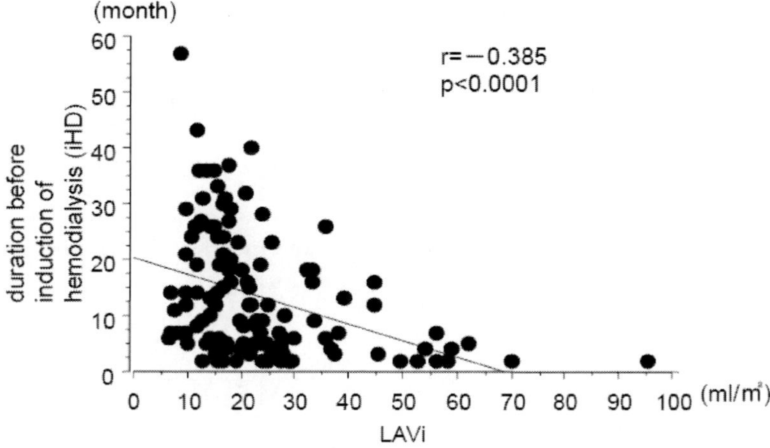

Figure 5. Correlation between duration before induction of hemodialysis (iHD) and left ventricular diastolic function (LAVi) in the diabetes group and in the nondiabetes group with CKD. As LA volume increases, duration before iHD decreases.

LVMI increased with decreasing renal function in CKD (stage 1–5) patients (Figure 6). In the univariate analysis, SBP, urine protein/urine creatinine ratio, serum creatinine, phosphorus, and erythropoietin dose were directly correlated with LVMI (p < 0.01). The levels of Hb, serum albumin, and Fe were inversely correlated with LVMI (p < 0.0001). In

     Hiroaki Io and Yasuhiko Tomino

stepwise linear regression analysis, SBP and Hb were identified as independent risk factors for LVMI (Table 2). The prevalence of LVH increased with advanced CKD (p < 0.001). The prevalence of LVH was 56.5% in the patients with CKD stage I, 52.2% in those with CKD stage II, 73.3% in those with CKD stage III, 81.3% in those with CKD stage IV, and 89.1% in those with CKD stage V. When the mean SBP and Hb with and without LVH in each CKD stag were compared, SBP was significantly higher in the patients with LVH in stages II and V and Hb was significantly lower in the patients with LVH in stages IV and V than in those in the other stages (Table 3).

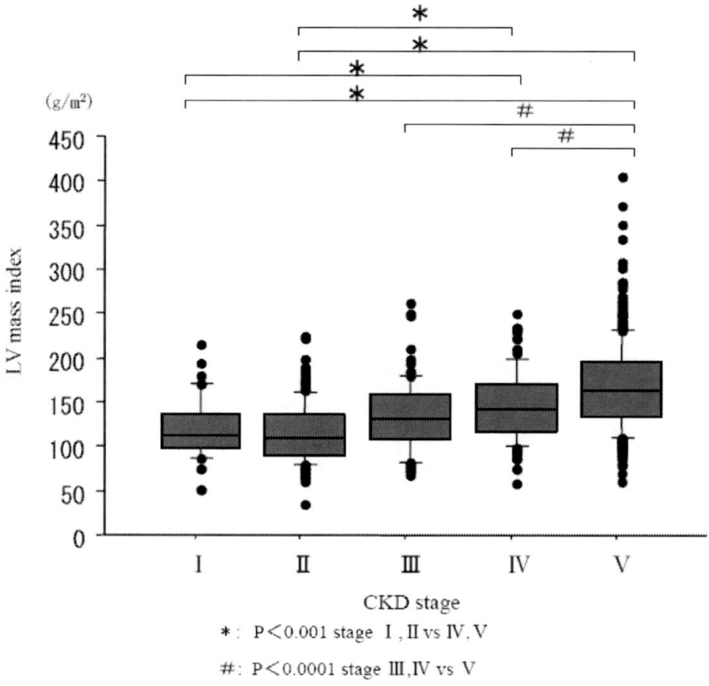

Figure 6. Comparison of LVMI among stages of CKD 1–5. LVMI is significantly higher in stages 4 and 5 than in stages 1 and 2 (p < 0.001).

Table 2. Stepwise linear regression analysis of factors associated with LVMI in CKD stage1-5

	P value	R value	F value
SBP	<0.0001	0.741	**36.74**
u-Pro/Cr	<0.0001	2.036	0.254
Alb	0.0045	-3.295	1.546
s-Cre	<0.0001	4.882	2.413
Hb	<0.0001	-7.808	**64.55**
EPO	<0.0001	0.001	1.829
Pi	<0.0001	8.214	0.169
Fe	0.0005	-0.190	1.068

Abbreviations: SBP: systolic BP, u-Pro/Cr:urine protein/urine creatinine ratio, Alb:albumin, s-Cre:serum concentration of creatinine, Hb:hemoglobin, EPO: Dose of erythropoietin /month, Pi:phosphorus, Fe: serum concentration of Fe.

Table 3. Cmparison of clinical paramenters with and without LVH in each CKD stages

	Without LVH	With LVH	p
CKD stage I	44%	57%	
Mean SBP (mmHg)	123.4 ± 19.3	132.0 ± 21.0	0.1642
Mean Hb (g/dL)	13.7 ± 1.9	14.1 ± 1.8	0.4822
CKD stage II	48%	52%	
Mean SBP (mmHg)	126.8 ± 21.5	138.0 ± 21.7	**0.0076**
Mean Hb (g/dL)	14.1 ± 1.7	13.7 ± 2.0	0.3787
CKD stage III	27%	73%	
Mean SBP (mmHg)	129.7 ± 19.6	139.4 ± 22.0	0.0648
Mean Hb (g/dL)	13.0 ± 1.9	12.5 ± 2.1	0.3152
CKD stage IV	19%	81%	
Mean SBP (mmHg)	134.2 ± 23.9	142.8 ± 22.2	0.1014
Mean Hb (g/dL)	12.6 ± 2.0	10.7 ± 2.1	**0.0002**
CKD stage V	11%	89%	
Mean SBP (mmHg)	131.2 ± 16.0	146.0 ± 19.8	**< 0.0001**
Mean Hb (g/dL)	9.5 ± 1.3	9.0 ± 1.4	**0.0139**

Data are shown as mean ± SD. LVH: left ventricular hypertrophy, BP: blood pressure.

4. CKD (Stages 1–5) Longitudinal Study

The rates of change of SBP and the urinary protein/creatinine ratio were significantly correlated with that of LVMI (Figure 7). The rates of change of Hb and estimated GFR were inversely correlated with that of LVMI (Figure 8).

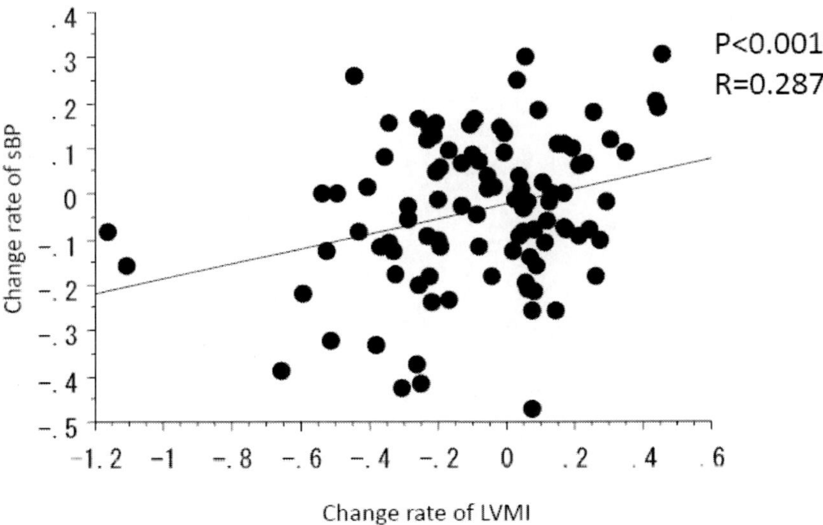

Figure 7. Correlation between rates of change of sBP and LVMI in CKD 1–5. The rate of change of sBP is significantly correlated with that of LVMI.

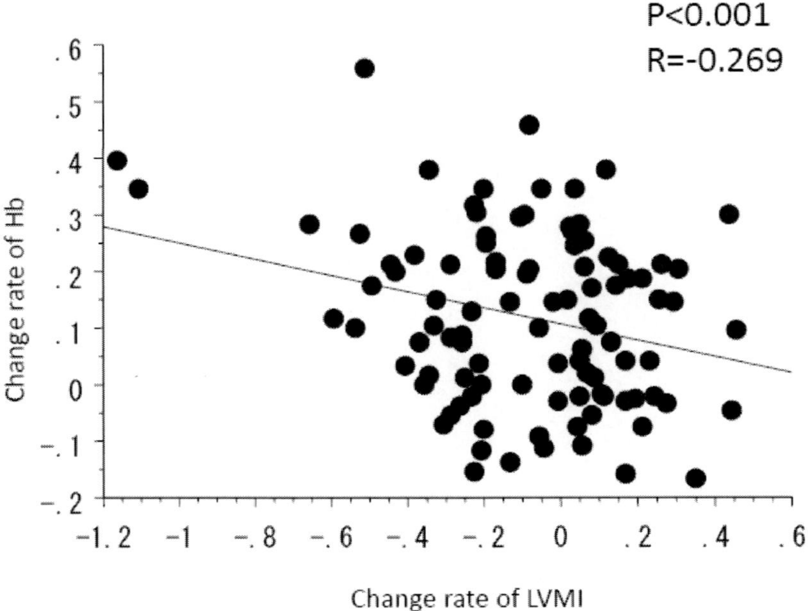

Figure 8. Correlation between rates of change of Hb and LVMI in CKD 1–5. The rate of change of Hb is inversely correlated with that of LVMI.

Table 4. Stepwise linear regression analysis of factors associated with change rate of LVMI for improvement group

Factors	P Value	R Value	F Value
Age (at baseline)	0.6821	0.063	---
Systolic blood pressure	**0.0046**	**0.415**	**8.938**
Diastolic blood pressure	0.1347	0.226	--
Urinary protein/u-creatinine	0.442	0.143	--
eGFR	0.121	0.240	--
Serum creatinine	0.5112	0.101	--
Serum albumin	0.9993	0.322	--
Hemoglobin	0.300	0.158	--
TSAT	0.9791	0.005	--
Serum calcium	0.9711	0.006	--
Serum phosphorus	0.5090	0.103	--
Serum iPTH	0.4894	0.221	--
Total cholesterol	0.9754	0.005	--
LDL cholesterol	0.2059	0.501	--
HDL cholesterol	0.5712	0.119	--

Abbreviations: LVMI, left ventricular mass index; eGFR, estimated glomerular filtration rate; iPTH, intact parathyroid hormone ; LDL, low density lipoprotein; HDL, high density lipoprotein; TSAT, transferin saturation; TIBC, total iron binding capacity.

Table 5. Stepwise linear regression analysis of factors associated with change rate of LVMI for worsening group

Factors	P Value	R Value	F Value
Age (at baseline)	0.4264	0.108	--
Systolic blood pressure	**0.0169**	**0.332**	**5.087**
Diastolic blood pressure	0.8915	0.019	--
Urinary protein/u-creatinine	**0.0057**	**0.416**	**8.595**
eGFR	0.0708	0.243	--
Serum creatinine	0.0943	0.226	--
Serum albumin	0.9088	0.016	--
Hemoglobin	**0.0160**	**−0.362**	**6.200**
TSAT	0.6187	0.088	--
Serum calcium	0.6042	0.071	--
Serum phosphorus	**0.0494**	**0.271**	2.423
Serum iPTH	0.3662	0.371	--
Total cholesterol	0.3429	0.138	--
LDL cholesterol	0.3972	0.349	--
HDL cholesterol	0.3670	0.202	--

Abbreviations: LVMI, left ventricular mass index; eGFR, estimated glomerular filtration rate; iPTH, intact parathyroid hormone ; LDL, low density lipoprotein; HDL, high density lipoprotein; TSAT, transferin saturation; TIBC, total iron binding capacity.

The rates of change of SBP and Hb were identified as independent risk factors for the rate of change of LVMI in the multivariate regression analysis. Table 3 shows the univariate analysis of factors associated with LVMI in the improvement group. The rate of change of SBP was significantly correlated with that of LVMI. Table 4 shows the results of the stepwise linear regression analysis of factors associated with LVMI in the worsening group. The rates of change of SBP, the urinary protein/creatinine ratio, and phosphorus were significantly correlated with that of LVMI, and the rate of change of Hb was inversely correlated with that of LVMI. The rates of change of SBP, urinary protein/creatinine ratio, and Hb were identified as independent risk factors for the rate of change of LVMI in the multivariate regression analysis.

Discussion

LVH is a common independent risk factor for cardiac death in CKD and ESKD patients. The prevalence and severity of LVH was increased in parallel with the severity of CKD. LVH is the most powerful indicator of mortality and cardiovascular complications in patients with CKD [15]. Our results showed that plasma ANP is one of the most important risk predictors of LVH [16]. The correlation between plasma ANP and LV mass in this study was comparable with that in previous studies [17, 18]. It has been hypothesized that LA size represents the integration of LV diastolic performance (compliance) over time. Thus, LA volume provides a long-term view of diastolic dysfunction, regardless of the loading conditions and filling pressure present at the time of examination [19]. A direct relationship between the transmitral flow velocity pattern and the plasma ANP level has not been previously reported in PD patients. In our study, the plasma ANP level showed a significant correlation with LAD and the peak A wave. These results suggest that the peak A wave is a potential indicator of excessive preload in PD patients. E wave or peak E/peak A and ANP level in our study were not related to the transmitral flow velocity pattern, which showed a diastolic dysfunction pattern [20].

Studies on hemodialysis patients without hypertension suggest that LVH may be related to certain factors, such as hyperparathyroidism, sympathetic activity, and reflection of the pulse wave, because of stiffened arteries and anemia [21-23]. Normalization of hemoglobin (13–14 g/dl) with recombinant human erythropoietin (rHuEpo) treatment did not induce regression of LV dilatation and concentric LVH [21]. On the other hand, treatment of renal anemia with rHuEpo improved cardiac performance and induced regression of LVH in one study [22]. In our study, the mean Hb level was significantly improved after initiation of HD and was maintained during the observation period. LVMI tended to decrease after 24 months. However, it was difficult to improve LVH in groups B and C (Figure 1). Comparable BP control between the groups might have decreased the potential development of LVH. In contrast, in patients who did achieve the protocol targets, changes in LVMI were consistent with the findings of previous studies that identified anemia as an independent predictor of LVH [23] and with changes in volume-based parameters that might be of particular importance as determinants of LV growth. Therefore, there is some evidence that the avoidance of anemia, together with control of BP and volume status, might favorably affect LV growth among patients with HD. Another study reported that normotensive HD patients showed no decrease in LVH for 2.5 years, although LAD increased [24]. The volume expansion may at least partially explain the persistence of or development of LVH. This finding is supported by studies on daily HD [25], a treatment modality that greatly facilitates volume control. In patients on nocturnal HD, there is a notable reduction in LVMI and LV function [26]. Total peripheral vascular resistance is decreased with endothelium-dependent vasodilatation restored [27]. Some, but not all, studies have demonstrated a decrease in erythropoietin requirements among patients converting from thrice- weekly HD to nocturnal HD [28, 29].

LA size is associated very strongly with LVH, and echocardiographic monitoring of LA size has recently emerged as an independent prognostic predictor of cardiovascular risk in patients with ESKD. In our study, there was a significant correlation with LA size and LVMI (p < 0.0001). We have recently demonstrated a significant correlation between LA volume index and LVMI in nondiabetic patients [30]. Age is an important determinant of arterial stiffness. Vascular aging occurs with advancing age and is associated with vascular wall changes, which can increase arterial stiffness. The receptor for advanced glycation end products link proteins increases arterial stiffness in diabetes and aging [31]. In our study, age was significantly correlated with LVMI.

The ectonucleotide pyrophosphatase phosphodiesterase 1 gene—a regulator of insulin sensitivity whose variability has been associated with insulin resistance (IR) in ESKD—and IR is also a relevant factor in the pathogenesis of LVH [32]. We also found that LVMI was larger in diabetic patients than in nondiabetic patients.

One study reported that serum phosphorus can stimulate phenotypic transformation of vascular smooth muscle cells into osteoblasts [33]. In our study, the level of serum phosphorus was significantly correlated with LVMI, and 25% of patients were on vitamin D treatment. LVH was present in 238 patients (55%) not on vitamin D therapy and in 94 patients (22%) on vitamin D therapy. The B allele of vitamin D receptor gene polymorphism may serve as a marker of altered vitamin D-signaling in ESRD patients and was independently related to LVH and LVH progression in ESRD patients [34].

We found that the prevalence of LVH was high, especially in CKD stages 4 and 5. There was a significant correlation between Hb and LVMI ($p < 0.05$) in stage 4 and between age, SBP, and LVMI ($p < 0.0001$) in stage 5. In addition, SBP and Hb were identified as independent risk factors associated with LVMI in the multivariate regression analysis. LVH might be a beneficial compensatory process in patients with CKD and allow the left ventricle to produce additional force to increase cardiac work and maintain constant wall tension. In our study, SBP was significantly higher and Hb was lower in patients with LVH than in patients without LVH, especially in CKD stages 4 and 5. Maintenance of SBP is predicted to have beneficial effects on the course of LVH. Fluid volume management and maintenance of a near euvolemic state are crucial for the amelioration of LVH [18, 35].

The rate of change of SBP was identified as an independent risk factor for changes in LVMI. Previous studies have shown that treatment of hypertension partially improves LV dilatation and LVH [36] [37]. Recently, it was reported that systolic arterial hypertension and elevated pulse pressure were closely associated with LVH in predialysis patients, which suggested that fluid overload and increased arterial stiffness have important roles in LVH well before starting dialysis therapy [38]. Thus, hypertension has been consistently associated with cardiovascular morbidity and LVH in CKD patients, and the results of our study are consistent with those in the literature. Maintaining low levels of SBP should have beneficial effects on the course of LVH in CKD patients [39].

The rate of change of Hb was identified as an independent risk factor for changes in LVMI. Anemia is considered to be one of the uremia-related factors associated with cardiovascular risk in patients with CKD [40], but few studies are available on the relationship between anemia and cardiovascular morbidity and mortality before starting dialysis treatment. Treatment of anemia improves survival, decreases morbidity and mortality, and increases quality of life in CKD patients. Partial elimination of anemia in patients with heart failure and CKD improves cardiac function [41]. Previously, it was reported that LVMI was reduced by increases in Hb [40, 42]. Our results were supported by findings of previous studies evaluating patients with CKD. However, recently the CHOIR study revealed that a targeted hemoglobin level of 13.5 g/dl was more harmful than 11.3 g/dl in predialysis patients with CKD and resulted in no incremental improvement in the quality of life [43]. In addition, the CREATE study showed that in patients with stage 3 or stage 4 CKD and mild-to-moderate anemia, normalization of hemoglobin levels in the range from 13.0 to 15.0 g/dl did not reduce cardiovascular events when compared with the use of a lower target range (10.5–11.5g/dl) [44]. Guidelines for treatment of anemia in CKD patients have existed since 1997 [45], but the optimal target Hb levels for patients with various stages of CKD are unclear. Following studies that did not provide support for these guidelines, the guidelines were revised in 2007 to reset the upper limit target value to 12 g/dl [46]. Evidence concerning the target value of anemia treatment of CKD patients is not sufficient, especially for the upper limit target value, and more studies are required. Moreover, it is thought that aggressive treatment is needed because the level of Hb did not reach the target value in our study (baseline 10.0 ± 2.2 mg/dl, follow-up period 9.5 ± 2.0 mg/dl). Our study showed that treatment of anemia should prevent LVH and progression of renal dysfunction [47].

There are some potential limitations to our study. It has a selection bias associated with its retrospective nature, and it was not a double-blinded study. Furthermore, because this is an observational study, it can only establish an association but not a causal relationship between SBP, Hb, and LVH. Another limitation is uncertainty about averaging 24-h home ambulatory BP monitoring and patient compliance during the use of antihypertensive medication prior to the examination. Finally, we did not perform cardiac magnetic resonance imaging, which, in the past 10 years, has become the new gold standard because of its high precision, reliability, and ability to measure LVMI [48]. This new method will certainly refine the relative role of LVM in the risk assessment of patients with ESKD. Future studies including this method are warranted to asses this.

Conclusion

Our results suggest recommendations and a possible algorithm to reduce LVH in dialysis patients. BP must be kept lower and Alb must be maintained, for example, by decreasing urinary protein before initiation of dialysis. SBP must be kept lower and plasma ANP must be decreased by controlling overhydration, and Hb levels must be maintained after initiation of HD. It is difficult to improve LVH in HD patients.

The left ventricular structure, contraction, and compliance were well preserved in PD patients undergoing aggressive treatment on the basis of plasma ANP and LAD measurements. It is important to treat hypertension, overhydration based on ANP, and anemia before initiation of dialysis. Our findings may have some therapeutic implications for strategies used to treat predialysis and dialysis patients.

Acknowledgments

We are indebted to the nephrologists (Drs. Masako Furukawa, Michiko Sato, Kozue Okumura, Mayumi Matsumoto, Nao Nohara : Division of Nephrology, Department of Internal Medicine, Juntendo University Faculty of Medicine, Tokyo, Japan) and the patients at the Juntendo University Hospital for their collaboration in this study.

Disclosures

None.

References

[1] Go AS, Chertow GM, Fan D, McCulloch CE, Hsu CY. Chronic kidney disease and the risk of death, cardiovascular events, and hospitalization. *N. Engl. J. Med.* 2004; 351: 1296-1305.

[2] Vanholder R, Massy Z, Argiles A, Spasovski G, Verbeke F, and Lameire N for the European Uremic Toxin Work Group. Chronic kidney disease as cause of cardiovascular morbidity and mortality. *Nephrol. Dial Transplant* 2005; 20: 1048-1056.

[3] Parfrey PS, Foley RN, Harnett JD, Kent GM, Murray DC, Barre PE. Outcome and risk factors for left ventricular disorders in chronic uraemia. *Nephrol Dial Transplant* 1996; 11: 1277-1285.

[4] Levin A, Singer J, Thompson CR, Ross H, Lewis M. Prevalent left ventricular hypertrophy in the predialysis population: identifying opportunities for intervention. *Am. J. Kidney Dis.* 1996; 27: 347-354.

[5] Sarnak MJ, Levey AS, Schoolwerth AC, et al. Kidney disease as a risk factor for development of cardiovascular disease. A statement from the American Heart Association Councils on Kidney in Cardiovascular Disease, High Blood Pressure Research, Clinical Cardiology, and Epidemiology and Prevention. *Circulation* 2003; 108: 2154-2169.

[6] Foley RN, Parfrey PS, Kent GN, Harnett JD, Murray DC, Barre PE. Long-term evolution of cardiomyopathy in dialysis patients. *Kidney International* 1998; 54: 1720-1725.

[7] Levy D, Garrison RJ, Savage DD, Kannel WB, Castelli WP. Prognostic implications of echocardiography determined left ventricular mass in the Framingham Heart Study. *N. Eng. J. Med.* 1990; 332: 1561-1566.

[8] Foley RN, Parfrey PS, Kent GM, Harnett JD, Murray DC, Barre PE. Serial change in echocardiographic parameters and cardiac failure in end-stage renal disease. *J. Am. Soc. Nephrol.* 2000; 11: 912-916.

[9] Jari AL, Sudhir K, Jaakko E, Matti H, Jukka TS. Left atrium size and the risk of cardiovascular death in middle-aged men. *Arch. Intern Med.* 2005; 165: 1788-1793.

[10] Takeichi N, Fukuda N, Tamura Y, Oki T, Ito S. Relationship between left atrium function and plasma level of atrial natriuretic peptide in patients with heart disease. *Cardiology* 1998; 90: 13-19.

[11] Lang RM, Bierig M, Devereux RB Flachskampf FA. Recommendations for chamber quantification: a report from the American Society of Echocardiography's Guidelines and Standards Committee and the Chamber Quantification Writing Group, developed in conjunction with the European Association of Echocardiography, a branch of the European Society of Cardiology. *J. Am. Soc. Echocardiogr* 2005; 18: 1440-1463.

[12] Devereux RB, Alonso DR, Lutas EM. Echocardiographic assessment of left ventricular hypertrophy. Comparison to necropsy findings. *Am. J. Cardiol.* 1986; 57: 450-458.

[13] Harnett JD, Murphy B, Collingwood P, Purchase L, Kent G, Parfrey PS. The reliability and validity of echocardiographic measurement of left ventricular mass index in hemodialysis patients. *Nephron* 1993; 65: 212-214.

[14] Sanfilippo AJ, Abascal VM, Sheehan M, Oertel LB, Harrigan P, Hughes RA, Weyman AE. Atrial enlargement as a consequence of atrial fibrillation. A prospective echocardiographic study. *Circulation*.1990; 82: 792-797.

[15] Middleton RJ, Parfrey PS, Foley RN. Left ventricular hypertrophy in the renal patient. *J. Am. Soc. Nephrol.* 2001; 40: 1079-84.

[16] Io H, Matsumoto M, Okumura K, Sato M, Masuda A, Furukawa M, Nohara N, Tanimoto M, Kodama F, Hagiwara S, Gohda T, Shimizu Y, Tomino Y. Predictive factors associated with left ventricular hypertrophy at baseline and in the follow-up period in non-diabetic hemodialysis patients. *Seminars in Dialysis* 2011; 24: 349-354.

[17] Nakatani T, Naganuma T, Masuda C et al. The prognostic role of atrial natriuretic peptides in hemodialysis patients. *Blood Purif* 2003; 21: 395-400.

[18] Io H, Ro Y, Sekiguchi Y, Shimaoka T, Inuma J, Hotta Y, Aruga S, Inami Y, Sato M, Kobayashi T, Masuda A, Kaneko K, Hamada C, Ohtaki E, Horikoshi S, Tomino Y. Cardiac function and structure in longitudinal analysis of echocardiography in peritoneal dialysis patients. *Peritoneal Dialysis International* 2010; 30: 353-361.

[19] Tsang TS, Barnes ME, Gersh BJ, et al. Prediction of risk for first age-related cardiovascular events in an elderly population: the incremental value of echocardiography. *J. Am. Coll Cardiol.* 2003; 42: 1199-1205.

[20] Tamura T, Kawaguchi Y, Tojou K, Ohta M, Sugimoto K, Hosoya T. Clinical usefulness of Doppler echocardiography for the assessment of dry weight in dialysis patients with known heart disease. *Jpn Soc. Dial Ther.* 2000; 33: 1409-1416.

[21] Foley RN, parfrey PS, Morgan J, et al. Effect of hemoglobin levels in hemodialysis patients with asymptomatic cardiomyopathy. *Kidney Int.* 2000; 58: 1325-1335.

[22] Jeren-Strujic B, Raos V, Jeren T, Horvatin-Godler S. Morphologic and functional changes of left ventricle in dialyzed patients after treatment with recombinant human erythropoietin (r-HuEPO). *Angiology* 2000; 51: 131-139.

[23] Levin A, Djurdjev O, Barrett B, Burgess E, Carlisle E, Ethier J, Jindal K, Mendelssohn D, Tobe S, Singer J, Thompson C. Cardiovascular disease in patients with chronic kidney disease: Getting to the heart of the matter. *Am. J. Kidney Dis.* 2001; 38: 1398-1407.

[24] Huting J, Kramer W, Schutterle G, Wizemann V. Analysis of left-ventricular changes associated with chronic hemodialysis. A noninvasive follow-up study. *Nephron* 1988; 49: 284-290.

[25] Fagugli RM, Reboldi G, Quintaliani G, et al. Short daily hemodialysis: blood pressure control and left ventricular mass reduction in hypertensive hemodialysis patients. *Am. J. Kidney Dis.* 2005; 38: 371-376.

[26] Chan CT, Floras JS, Miller JA, Richardson RMA, Pierratos A. Regression of left ventricular hypertrophy after conversion to nocturnal hemodialysis. *Kidney Int.* 2002; 61:2235-2239.

[27] Chan CT, Harvey PJ, Picton P, Pierratos A, Miller JA, Floras JS. Short-term blood pressure, noradrenergic, and vascular effects of nocturnal home hemodialysis. *Hypertension* 2003; 42: 925-931.

[28] Schwartz DI, Pierratos A, Richardson RM, Fentos SS, Chan CT. Impact of nocturnal home hemodialysis on anemia management in patients with end stage renal disease. *Clin. Nephrol.* 2005; 63: 202-208.

[29] Rao M, Muirhead N, Klarenbach S, Moist L, Lindsay RM. Management of anemia with quotidian hemodialysis. *Am. J. Kidney Dis.* 2003; 42: 18-23.

[30] Furukawa M, Io H, Tanimoto M, Hagiwara S, Horikoshi S, Tomino T. Predictive Factors Associated with the Period of Time before Initiation of Hemodialysis in CKD Stages 4 and 5. *Nephron Clin. Pract.* 2011; 117: c341-c347.

[31] Jani B, Rajkumar C. Ageing and vascular ageing. *Postgrad med. J.* 2006; 82: 357-362.

[32] Spoto B, Testa A, Parlongo RM, Tripepi G, Trischitta V, Mallamaci F, Zoccali C. Iinsulin resistance and left ventricular hypertrophy in end-stage renal disease: association between the ENNP1 gene and left ventricular concentric remodeling. *Nephrol. Dial Transplant.* 2011; 0: 1-6.

[33] Moe SM, Duan D, Doehle BP, O'Neill KD, Chen NX. Uremia induces the osteoblast differentiation factor Cbfal in human blood vessels. *Kidney Int.* 2003; 63: 1003-1011.

[34] Testa A, Mallamaci F, Benedetto FA, Pisano A, Tripepi G, Malatino L, Thadhani R, Zoccali C. Vitamin D Receptor (VDR) gene polymorphism is associated with left ventricular (LV) mass and predicts left ventricular hypertrophy (LVH) progression in end-stage renal disease (ESRD) patients. *J. Bone Miner Res.* 2010; 25: 313-319.

[35] Guyton AC, Coleman TG, Wilcox CS. Quantitative analysis of the pathophysiology of hypertension. *J. Am. Soc. Nephrol.* 1999; 10: 2248-2249.

[36] London GM, Pannier B, Guerin AP, Marchais SJ, Safar ME, Cuche JL. Cardiac hypertrophy, aortic compliance, peripheral resistance, and wave reflection in end-stage renal disease: Comparative effects of ACE inhibition and calcium channel blockade. *Circulation* 1994; 90: 2786-2796.

[37] Cannella G, Paoletti E, Delfino R, Peloso G, Rolla D, Molinari S. Prolonged therapy with ACE inhibitors induces a regression of left ventricular hypertrophy of dialyzed uremic patients independently from hypotensive effects. *Am. J. Kidney Dis.* 1997; 30: 659-664.

[38] Paoletti E, Bellino D, Cassoottana P, Rolla D, Cannella G. Left ventricular hypertrophy in nondiabetic predialysis CKD. *Am. J. Kidney Dis.* 2005; 46: 320-327.

[39] Matsumoto M, Io H, Furukawa M, Okumura K, Masuda A, Seto T, Takagi M, Sato M, Nagahama L, Omote K, Hisada A, Horikoshi S, Tomino Y. Risk factors associated with increased left ventricular mass index in chronic kidney disease patients evaluated using echocardiography. *J. Nephrol.* 2012; 25: 794-801.

[40] Portoles J, Torralbo A, Martin P, Rodrigo J, Herrero JA, Barrientos A. Cardiovascular effects of recombinant human erythropoietin in predialysis patients. *Am. J. Kidney Dis.* 1997; 29: 541-548.

[41] Silverberg DS, Wexler D, Blum M, et al. The use of subcutaneous erythropoietin and intravenous iron for the treatment of the anemia of severe, resistant congestive heart failure improves cardiac and renal function and functional cardiac class, and markedly reduces hospitalization. *J. Am. Coll Cardiol.* 2000; 35: 1737-1744.

[42] Hayashi T, Suzuki A, Shoji T, Togawa M, Okada N, Tsubakihara Y, Imai E, Hori M. Cardiovascular effect of normalizing the hematocrit level during erythropoietin therapy in predialysis patients with chronic renal failure. *Am. J. Kidney Dis.* 2000; 35: 250-256.

[43] Singh AK, Szczech L, Tang KL, Barnhart H, Sapp S, Wolfson M, Reddan D (CHOIR Investigators). Correction of anemia with epoetin alpha in chronic kidney disease. *N. Engl. J. Med.* 2006; 355: 2085-2098.

[44] Drüeke TB, Locatelli F, Clyne N, Eckardt KU, Macdougall IC, Tsakiris D, Burger HU, Scherhag A (CREATE Investigators). Normalization of hemoglobin level in patients with chronic kidney disease and anemia. *N. Engl. J. Med.* 2006; 355: 2071-2084.

[45] National Kidney Foundation-Dialysis Outcomes Quality Initiative. NKF-DOQI clinical practice guidelines for the treatment of anemia of chronic renal failure. *Am. J. Kidney Dis.* 1997; 30: S192-240.

[46] National Kidney Foundation. K/DOQI clinical practice guideline and clinical practice recommendations for anemia in chronic kidney disease: update of hemoglobin target. *Am. J. Kidney Dis.* 2007; 50: 471-530.

[47] Okumura K, Io H, Matsumoto M, Seto T, Takagi M, Masuda A, Furukawa M, Nagahama L, Omote K, Hisada A, Hamada C, Horikoshi S, Tomino Y. Predictive factors associated with change rates of LV hypertrophy and renal dysfunction in CKD patients. *Clin. Nephrol.* 2013; 79: 7-14.

[48] Aqabiti RE, Muiesan ML, Salvetti M. New approaches to the assessment of left ventricular hypertrophy. *Ther. Adv. Cardiovasc. Dis.* 2007; 1: 119-128.

In: Left Ventricular Hypertrophy (LVH)
Editor: Richard T. Matthews

ISBN: 978-1-63463-022-1
© 2015 Nova Science Publishers, Inc.

Chapter 7

Insights from Metabolomic Analyses of Left Ventricular Hypertrophy and Heart Failure

Takao Kato[*]
Cardiovascular Center, Tazuke Kofukai Medical Research Institute,
Kitano Hospital, Japan

Abstract

Left ventricular hypertrophy (LVH) accompanies the altered energy metabolism of the heart, and the altered energetics is hypothesized to play an important role in the progression of heart failure. However, the mechanism underlying these changes, and whether these changes are beneficial or detrimental, are not known because simultaneous evaluation of multiple metabolites is difficult and substrates in perfusion buffer are limited in ex vivo perfused heart experiments. Metabolomics is an emerging field of study, which uses mass spectrometry and/or nuclear magnetic resonance. This enables the monitoring of hundreds of metabolites from tissues or body fluids, and facilitates the identification of various metabolites simultaneously, and helps evaluate global changes in metabolites levels during cellular and physiological responses to external stimuli. The metabolomic analysis of an animal model with hypertensive LVH and decompensated heart failure indicates significant changes in cardiac energy metabolism. In human studies, metabolomics has been used to analyze blood or heart tissue samples from patients with cardiovascular diseases, such as ischemic heart disease, atrial fibrillation, ischemia reperfusion, heart failure, and metabolic syndrome. These reports not only provide significant information on the underlying mechanism of these diseases but also suggest potential biomarkers for the diagnosis of these conditions. Coupling metabolomics with other approaches, such as functional genomics and proteomics, can help determine the pathophysiology of cardiovascular diseases, discover biomarkers, and identify targets for therapeutic intervention.

[*] Address correspondence to:Takao Kato, M.D., Ph.D. Cardiovascular Center, Tazuke Kofukai Medical Research Institute, Kitano Hospital, Japan, TEL: +81-6-6312-8831; FAX: +81-6-6312-8867, Full institutional mailing addresses: 2-2-20 Ogimachi, Kita-ku, Osaka 530-8480, Japan, E-mail: takao-kato@kitano-hp.or.jp.

Keywords: Metabolomics analysis, left ventricular hypertrophy, heart failure

Introduction

The heart produces and consumes more energy than any other organ in the human body; the mechanism that facilitates the homeostasis of energy metabolism in heart has attracted the attention of many cardiologists and scientists. Left ventricular hypertrophy and systolic heart failure (HF) is a complex clinical syndrome that arises as a result of abnormalities in cardiac structure and/or function that impair the ability of the left ventricle to pump blood [1]. Left ventricular hypertrophy (LVH) is accompanied with an altered energy metabolism of the heart, and this alteration is hypothesized to play an important role in the progression of heart failure [2-4]. The hearts of dilated cardiomyopathy patients showed a shift towards greater glucose and lower fatty acid oxidation [5]. Carvedilol treatment increased cardiac uptake of ^{18}F-fluorodeoxyglucose and facilitated the improvement of cardiac function [6]. Moreover, inhibitors of fatty acid oxidation such as, trimetazidine, perhexiline, and etoxomir improved left ventricular function in patients [7-10].

However, whether these metabolic changes are beneficial or detrimental is not known [2]; moreover, the underlying mechanisms of these changes remain unelucidated because the simultaneous evaluation of multiple metabolites is difficult and substrates in perfusion buffer in *ex vivo* perfused heart experiments are limited. Therefore, using metabolomics, which is an emerging field that uses mass spectrometry and/or nuclear magnetic resonance, it is possible to monitor hundreds of metabolites from tissues or body fluids [11-13]. This facilitates the simultaneous identification of various metabolites, and helps evaluate global changes in metabolites levels during cellular and physiological responses to external stimuli. Thus, metabolomics can be a useful tool for evaluating the complex underlying mechanism of altered energetics in LVH and heart failure.

Analysis of Animal Models

Metabolomics has been successfully applied to animal models of cardiovascular diseases. The models that have been previously employed include those of systolic heart failure induced by environmental factors, tachycardia, myocardial infarction, and hypertension (Table 1). Combined with genetic manipulations using genetically engineered animals, metabolomics can clarify the role of a molecule of interest in a comprehensive manner. A combined metabolomics and proteomics analysis of heart tissue has been reported previously.

Here we present a differential metabolomics approach that utilizes capillary electrophoresis time-of-flight mass spectrometry to investigate the role of glycolysis and glucose oxidation as a new therapeutic target [14].We analyzed the cardiac energy metabolism of Dahl salt-sensitive (DS) rats fed on a high salt diet, which showed a distinct transition from compensated LV hypertrophy (LVH) to systolic heart failure [15]. DS rats fed a low salt diet were used as controls. *In situ* [31]P MR spectroscopy analysis indicated that the Phosphocreatine (PCr) /ATP ratio was decreased by 12% in the LVH stage and 42% in the heart failure stage (Figure 1).

Table 1. Metabolomic analysis of animal models of cardiovascular diseases

Type of intervention	Sample	Method	Number*	Changes in metabolites	Finding
Environmental model					
systolic HF (tachycardia-induced) [17]	Heart tissue	NMR	9/21	Increased; ADP+ATP, alanine, glucose, glutamate, taurine, etc. Decreased; alpha-ketoisoisovalerate.	Shift from glycolysis to α-ketoacid metabolism
MI [18]	Blood	GC-MS	24/N.D.	Increased; lactate, succinate, malate, phosphate, glycine, oxoproline, phenylalanine, proline, palmitate, etc.	IHD biomarkers
systolic HF (hypertension) [14]	Heart tissue	CE-MS	19/114	Increased; pyruvate, NADPH, GSH, GSSG. Decreased; alanine, succinate, $NADP^+$.	Pentose phosphate pathway activated
systolic HF (doxorubicin-induced) [19]	Heart tissue	NMR	3/15	Increased; acetate, succinate. Decreased; branched amino acids.	Biomarkers of doxorubicin toxicity
Normal heart [20]	Heart tissue	MLDI-TOF/TOF-MS	285	N.D.	Verification of the method
LVH (obesity) [21]	Heart tissue	NMR	N.D./22	Increased; unsaturated lipids. Decreased; glutamine/glutamate ratio	Several specific kinetic molecular patterns as a prelude to systolic HF
PPARγ agonist to obese rat [22]	Heart tissue	GC-MS	N.D.	Increased; cardiolipin. Decreased; free fatty acids.	Relationship between cardiolipin and PPARγ activation
Genetically Engineered model					
Angiotensin II [23]	Heart tissue	GC-MS	112/247	Increased; hypoxanthine, ketogenic animo acids (tyrosine, lysine, ornithine). Decreased; octanoic, oleic and linoleic acids.	Mitochondrial dysfunction in Ang2-induced hypertrophy
PKCϵ [24]	Heart tissue	NMR	9/23	Increased; choline, glutamate, adenosine. Decreased; glucose, lactate, glutamine, creatine.	PKCϵ may be protective by modulating glucose metabolism

Table 1. (Continued)

Type of intervention	Sample	Method	Number*	Changes in metabolites	Finding
ADH2 [25]	Heart tissue	CE-MS (fluxosome)	10/13	Increased; labeled intermediate metabolites of the glycolysis and pentose phosphate pathways	Glycolysis and pentose phosphate pathway activated by impaired ADH2 activity
PPARα [26]	Heart tissue	NMR, GC-MS, LC-MS	N.D.	Increased; lactate, mannitol, glycerophosphoric acid, adenosine. Decreased; alanine, glucose, glutamine, creatinine, fructose, proline, isocitrate, oxalic acid	Failure in glycolysis, Krebs-cycle, and gluconeogenesis
Dystrophin, MLP [27]	Heart tissue	NMR	9/28	taurine, lactate, phosphocholine, choline,creatine, glucose, citrate, lysine, alanine	Significant strain background effect. Change of metabolic profile still detectable in mutant mice.

MI; myocardial infarction, PKCε; protein kinase C epsilon, ADH2; aldehyde dehydrogenase 2, MLP; muscle LIM protein, Scn; cardiac sodium channel. MLDI-TOF time-of-flight, NADPH; reduced-form of nicotinamide adenine dinucleotide phosphate, NADP+; oxidized-form of nicotinamide adenine dinucleotide phosphate, GSH; reduced glutathione, GSSG; oxidized glutathione, *; number of metabolites changed/number of metabolites examined, N.D.; not determined.

Table 2. Metabolomic analysis of human cardiovascular diseases

Disease	Sample	Method	Number*	Changes in metabolites changed	Finding
systolic HF with depression [28]	Blood	GC-MS, LC-MS	154/423	Increased; several amino acids and dicarboxylic fatty acids	Neurotransmitter systems and fatty acid metabolism associate with depressed state.
Atherosclerosis [29]	Atherosclerotic plaque	NMR	1/10	Increased; taurine	Taurine may be increased to scavenge leukocyte derived free radicals
MI [31]	Blood	LC-MS	18/185	Metabolites related to pyrimidine metabolism, Krebs-cycle, and pentose phosphate pathway changed.	Metabolic profiling may be useful for early detection of myocardial infarction.
IHD and systolic HF [31]	Blood (coronary sinus)	MSx MS	N.D./63	Global suppression of metabolic fuel uptake in CHF. Elution of acylcarnitine, 3-hydroxybutyl-carnitine, and alanine increased.	Impaired Krebs-cycle function in systolic HF.
IHD[5] [32]	Blood	GC-MS	9/21	Several fatty acids	Several fatty acids may serve as biomarkers of IHD.
AF [33]	Heart tissue	NMR	3/21	Increased:β-hydroxybutyrate, fumarate, tyrosine	Ketone metabolism may be important in AF.
IHD [34]	Blood	NMR	N.D./6	N.D.	Metabolomic profile may detect IHD.
IHD[35]	Blood	NMR	N.D.	N.D.	NMR spectra pattern is weak in detecting IHD.
IHD [36]	Blood	LC-MS	23/171	γ-aminobutyric acid, oxaloacetate, citrulline, argininosuccinate, uric acid, citric acid	Metabolites of Krebs-cycle changed in sera from IHD patients.

HF; heart failure, MI; myocardial infarction, IHD;ischemic heart disease, AF; atrial fibrillation, *; number of metabolites changed/number of metabolites examined, GC; gas chromatography, MS; mass spectrometry, NMR; nuclear magnetic resonance, LC; liquid chromatography, N.D.; not determined.

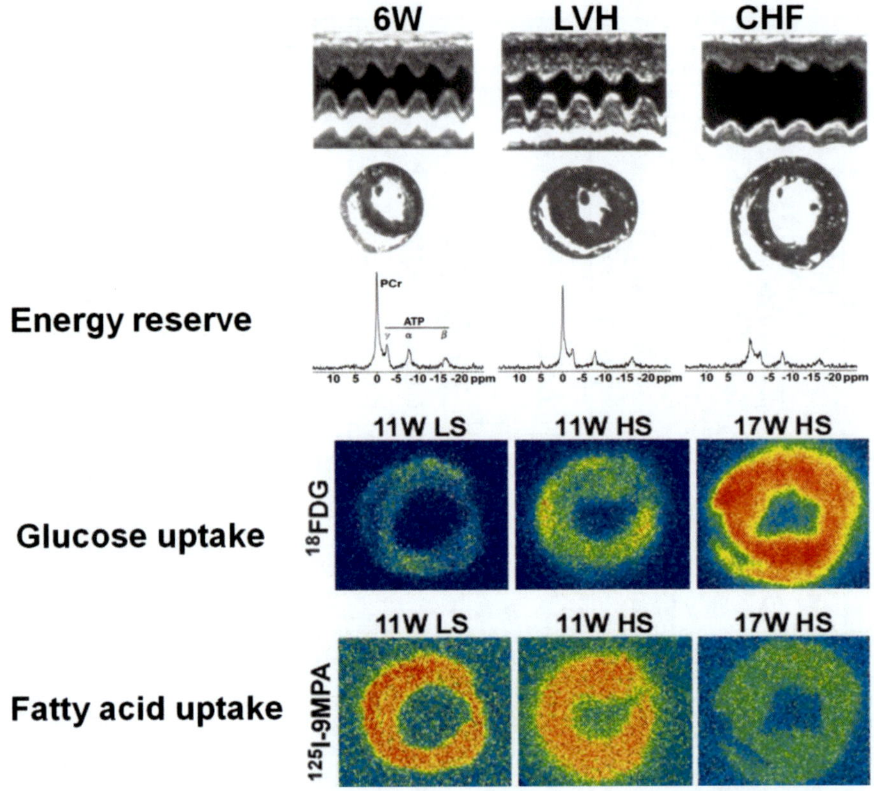

Figure 1. Metabolic remodeling in left ventricular hypertrophy (LVH) and congestive heart failure (CHF). Inbred male Dahl salt-sensitive (DS) rats were fed an 8% high-salt (HS) diet, which induced a distinct transition from compensated left ventricular hypertrophy to CHF. DS rats fed with low-salt diet (LS) were used as controls. In that model, the energy reserves assessed by Phosphocreatine (PCr)/ATP ratio were decreased by 12% in the LVH stage and 42% in the CHF stage. The uptake of [18]FDG, a glucose analogue, was increased by 1.4-fold in the LVH stage and by 2.4-fold in the CHF stage. The uptake of [125]I-9MPA, a fatty acid analogue, was not changed in the LVH stage but decreased by 36% in the CHF stage.

The uptake of ^{18}F-Fludeoxyglucose ([18]FDG), a glucose analogue, was increased by 1.4-fold in the LVH stage and by 2.4-fold in the heart failure stage. The uptake of [125]I-15-(*p*-iodophenyl)-9-*R*,*S*-methylpentadecanoic acid ([125]I-9MPA), a fatty acid analogue, was not changed in the LVH stage but decreased by 36% in the heart failure stage (Figure 1). The shift of substrate uptake from fatty acids to glucose was associated with decreased mRNA of fatty acid transporter and increased mRNA of glucose transporter (GLUT1). The gene expression related to glycolysis, fatty acid oxidation, and mitochondrial function was preserved in the LVH stage and was decreased in the heart failure stage, and was associated with decreases in protein expression levels of transcriptional regulators (Hypoxia-inducible factor-1α, peroxisome proliferator–activated receptor-γ coactivator-1-α, and peroxisome proliferator–activated receptor-α). A comprehensive analysis of the metabolome indicated a distinct change in metabolites related to glycolysis and the Krebs (TCA) cycle during the transition (Figure 2 and 3). Particularly, the pentose phosphate pathway that regulates the cellular redox state was found to be activated in the heart failure stage (Figure 3).

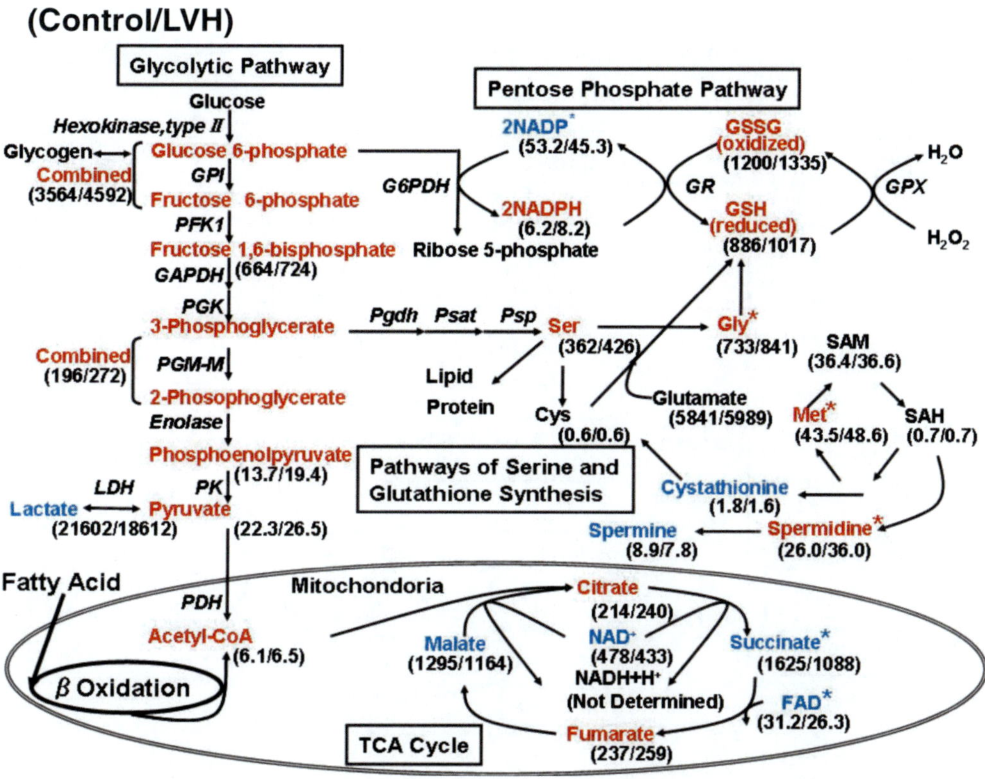

Figure 2. A comparison of metabolic profile between control and hypertrophy. The map illustrates glycolysis, pentose phosphate, Krebs (TCA)cycle, and serine and glutathione synthesis pathways. Red and blue indicate more than 5% increase and decrease in LVH compared to control, respectively. Results are expressed as control/ hypertrophy (n=4 for each group).*P<0.05 vs Control group.

Dichloroacetate (DCA), a compound known to enhance glucose oxidation, increased the energy reserve and [18]FDG uptake. DCA improved cardiac function and survival of animals, and decreased myocardial fibrosis and plasma brain natriuretic peptides levels. DCA augmented the activation of pentose phosphate pathway in congestive heart failure rats and decreased oxidative stress.

DCA also decreased the generation of oxidative stress and prevented the induction of cell death by hydrogen peroxide in cultured cardiomyocytes [14].

It is important to note that most of the changes in cardiac energy metabolism occurred at significant levels in the congestive heart failure stage, andalmost of these changes started in the LVH stage.

In addition, the substrate uptake or energy reserves decreased in the LVH stage. In conclusion, the transition from LVH to systolic heart failure is associated with a distinct change in the metabolic profile of heart. DCA attenuated the transition associated with increased energy reserves, as well as activation of the pentose phosphate pathway and reduced oxidative stress [16].

This study suggests that altered energetics is both a consequence and one of the causes of the transition from LVH to congestive heart failure, because targeting the altered energetics improved survival of rats with heart failure [14, 16].

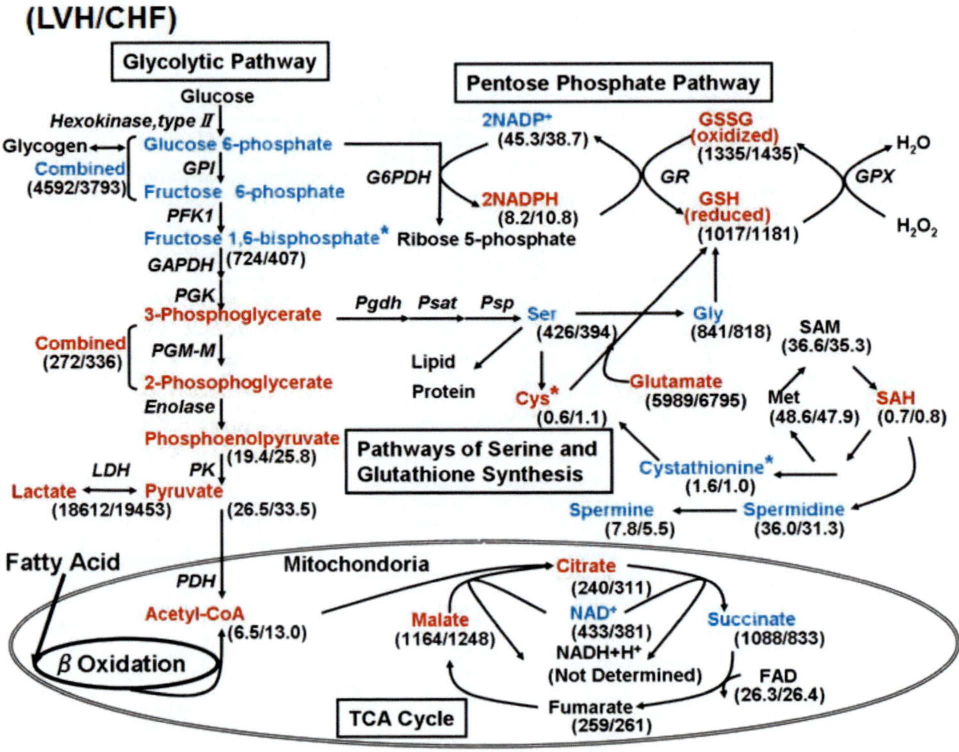

Figure 3. A comparison between the metabolic profile of hypertrophy and heart failure. The former part of metabolites of the glycolytic pathway are decreased, despite increase of the latter part of metabolites of glycolysis, NADPH, and GSH. Red and blue indicate more than 5% increase and decrease in LVH compared to control, respectively. Results are expressed as control/ hypertrophy (n=4 for each group).*P<0.05 vs LVH group.

Applications in Humans

The pathogenesis of several cardiovascular diseases, such as ischemic heart diseases, atrial fibrillation, ischemia reperfusion, systolic heart failure, and metabolic syndrome has been analyzed through metabolomics approaches, which in turn provided significant information. However, there are no reports of metabolomics analysis in patients with diastolic HF with normal ejection fraction. Samples from heart tissue and blood have been used in previous studies (Table 2). Analyses of human heart or vascular tissue, where metabolomic and proteomic approaches were used in combination, have also been reported. These reports identified useful biomarkers for diseases and/or provided new insights for understanding the pathogenesis of diseases.

However, applications in humans may be limited due to inter-individual variability. Studies which identify novel disease-related pathways are also restricted by the inherent unpredictability of the onset of pathological states. In addition, potential clinical confounders, such as diet or drug, watching as well as age, gender, circadian rhythm, and comorbidities can affect the results [11-13].

Conclusion

A metabolomics analysis can not only reveal significant information about the underlying mechanism of diseases but also identify potential biomarkers. The coupling of metabolomics with other approaches, such as functional genomics and proteomics, promises to shed new light on the pathophysiology of cardiovascular diseases, discovery of biomarkers, and identification of targets for therapeutic intervention.

Funding Sources

This work was supported by grants from the Japan Society for the Promotion of Science, the Suzuken Memorial Foundation, the Uehara Memorial Foundation, and the Tazuke Kofukai Medical Research Institutes.

References

[1]   Jessup M, Brozena S. (2003). Heart failure. *N. Engl. J. Med.* 348:2007-2018.

[2]   Ingwall JS. (2002) ATP and the heart. Kluwer academic publishers.

[3]   Stanley WC, Recchia FA, Lopaschuk GD. (2005). Myocardial substrate metabolism in the normal and failing heart. *Physiol. Rev.* 85:1093-1129.

[4]   Neubauer S. (2007). The failing heart-an engine out of fuel. *N. Engl. J. Med.* 356:1140-1151.

[5]   Davila-Roman VG, Vedala G, Herrero P, de las Fuentes L, Rogers JG, Kelly DP, Gropler RJ. (2002). Altered myocardial fatty acid and glucose metabolism in idiopathic dilated cardiomyopathy. *J. Am. Coll. Cardiol.* 40:271-277.

[6]   Wallhaus TR, Taylor M, DeGrado TR, Russell DC, Stanko P, Nickles RJ, Stone CK. (2001). Myocardial free fatty acid and glucose use after carvedilol treatment in patients with congestive heart failure. *Circulation.* 103:2441-2446.

[7]   Vitale C1, Wajngaten M, Sposato B, Gebara O, Rossini P, Fini M, Volterrani M, Rosano GM. (2004). Trimetazidine improves left ventricular function and quality of life in elderly patients with coronary artery disease. *Eur. Heart J.* 25:1814-821.

[8]   Lee L, Campbell R, Scheuermann-Freestone M, Taylor R, Gunaruwan P, Williams L, Ashrafian H, Horowitz J, Fraser AG, Clarke K, Frenneaux M. (2005). Metabolic modulation with perhexiline in chronic heart failure: a randomized, controlled trial of short-term use of a novel treatment. *Circulation.* 112:3280-3288.

[9]   Di Napoli P, Taccardi AA, Barsotti A. (2005). Long term cardioprotective action of trimetazidine and potential effect on the inflammatory process in patients with ischaemic dilated cardiomyopathy. *Heart.* 91:161-165.

[10]   Schmidt-Schweda S, Holubarsch C. (2000). First clinical trial with etomoxir in patients with chronic congestive heart failure. *Clin. Sci.* (Lond).99:27-35.

[11]   Lewis GD, Asnani A, Gerszten RE. (2008). Application of metabolomics to cardiovascular biomarker and pathway discovery. *J. Am. Coll. Cardiol.* 52:117-123.

[12] Nicholson JK, Lindon JC. (2008). Systems biology: *Metabonomics*. *Nature* 455:1054-1056.

[13] Mayr M. (2008). Metabolomics: ready for the prime time? *Circ. Cardiovasc. Genet.* 1:58-65.

[14] Kato T, Niizuma S, Inuzuka Y, Kawashima T, Okuda J, Tamaki Y, Iwanaga Y, Narazaki M, Matsuda T, Soga T, Kita T, Kimura T, Shioi T. (2010). Analysis of Metabolic Remodeling in Compensated Left Ventricular Hypertrophy and Heart Failure. *Circ. Heart Fail* 3:420-430.

[15] Inoko M, Kihara Y, Morii I, Fujiwara H, Sasayama S. (1994). Transition from compensatory hypertrophy to dilated, failing left ventricles in Dahl salt-sensitive rats. *Am. J. Physiol.* 267:H2471–H2482.

[16] Doenst T, Nguyen TD, Abel ED. (2013). Cardiac metabolism in heart failure: Implications beyond ATP production. *Circulation Research*.113:709-724.

[17] De Souza AI, Cardin S, Wait R, Chung YL, Vijayakumar M, Maguy A, Camm AJ, Nattel S. (2010). Proteomic and metabolomic analysis of atrial profibrillatory remodelling in congestive heart failure. *J. Mol. Cell. Cardiol* 49:851-863.

[18] Yao H, Shi P, Zhang L, Fan X, Shao Q, Cheng Y. (2010). Untargeted metabolic profiling reveals potential biomarkers in myocardial infarction and its application. *Mol. Biosyst.* 6:1061-1070.

[19] Andreadou I, Papaefthimiou M, Zira A, Constantinou M, Sigala F, Skaltsounis AL, Tsantili-Kakoulidou A, Iliodromitis EK, Kremastinos DT, Mikros E.(2009). Metabonomic identification of novel biomarkers in doxorubicin cardiotoxicity and protective effect of the natural antioxidant oleuropein. *NMR Biomed* 22:585-592.

[20] Sun G, Yang K, Zhao Z, Guan S, Han X, Gross RW. (2007). Shotgun metabolomics approach for the analysis of negatively charged water-soluble cellular metabolites from mouse heart tissue. *Anal. Chem.* 79:6629-6640.

[21] Roncalli J, Smih F, Desmoulin F, Dumonteil N, Harmancey R, Hennig S, Perez L, Pathak A, Galinier M, Massabuau P, Malet-Martino M, Senard JM, Rouet P. (2007). NMR and cDNA array analysis prior to heart failure reveals an increase of unsaturated lipids, a glutamine/glutamate ratio decrease and a specific transcriptome adaptation in obese rat heart. *J. Mol. Cell. Cardiol.* 42:526-539.

[22] Watkins SM, Reifsnyder PR, Pan HJ, German JB, Leiter EH. (2002). Lipid metabolome-wide effects of the PPARgamma agonist rosiglitazone. *J. Lipid Res.* 43:1809-1817.

[23] Mervaala E, Biala A, Merasto S, Lempiainen J, Mattila I, Martonen E, Eriksson O, Louhelainen M, Finckenberg P, Kaheinen P, Muller DN, Luft FC, Lapatto R, Oresic M.(2010). Metabolomics in angiotensin II-induced cardiac hypertrophy. *Hypertension*55:508-515.

[24] Mayr M, Liem D, Zhang J, Li X, Avliyakulov NK, Yang JI, Young G, Vondriska TM, Ladroue C, Madhu B, Griffiths JR, Gomes A, Xu Q, Ping P. (2009).Proteomic and metabolomic analysis of cardioprotection: Interplay between protein kinase C epsilon and delta in regulating glucose metabolism of murine hearts. *J. Mol. Cell. Cardiol.* 46:268-277.

[25] Endo J, Sano M, Katayama T, Hishiki T, Shinmura K, Morizane S, Matsuhashi T, Katsumata Y, Zhang Y, Ito H, Nagahata Y, Marchitti S, Nishimaki K, Wolf AM, Nakanishi H, Hattori F, Vasiliou V, Adachi T, Ohsawa I, Taguchi R, Hirabayashi Y,

Ohta S, Suematsu M, Ogawa S, Fukuda K.(2009). Metabolic remodeling induced by mitochondrial aldehyde stress stimulates tolerance to oxidative stress in the heart. *Circ. Res.* 105:1118-1127.

[26] Atherton HJ, Bailey NJ, Zhang W, Taylor J, Major H, Shockcor J,Clarke K, Griffin JL. (2006). A combined 1H-NMR spectroscopy-and mass spectrometry-based metabolomic study of the PPAR-alpha null mutant mouse defines profound systemic changes in metabolism linked to the metabolic syndrome. *Physiol. Genomics* 27:178-186.

[27] Wilding JR, Schneider JE, Sang AE, Davies KE, Neubauer S, Clarke K. (2005). Dystrophin- and MLP-deficient mouse hearts: marked differences in morphology and function, but similar accumulation of cytoskeletal proteins. *FASEB J.* 19:79-81..

[28] Steffens DC, Wei J, Krishnan KR, Karoly ED, Mitchell MW, O'Connor CM, Kaddurah-Daouk R. (2010). Metabolomic differences in heart failure patients with and without major depression. *J. Geriatr. Psychiatry Neurol.* 23:138-146.

[29] Mayr M, Grainger D, Mayr U, Leroyer AS, Leseche G, Sidibe A Herbin O, Yin X, Gomes A, Madhu B, Griffiths JR, Xu Q, Tedgui A, Boulanger CM.(2009). Proteomics, metabolomics, and immunomics on microparticles derived from human atherosclerotic plaques. *Circ. Cardiovasc. Genet.* 2:379-388.

[30] Lewis GD1, Wei R, Liu E, Yang E, Shi X, Martinovic M, Farrell L, Asnani A, Cyrille M, Ramanathan A, Shaham O, Berriz G, Lowry PA, Palacios IF, Taşan M, Roth FP, Min J, Baumgartner C, Keshishian H, Addona T, Mootha VK, Rosenzweig A, Carr SA, Fifer MA, Sabatine MS, Gerszten RE. (2008). Metabolite profiling of blood from individuals undergoing planned myocardial infarction reveals early markers of myocardial injury. *J. Clin. Invest.* 118:3503-3512.

[31] Turer AT, Stevens RD, Bain JR, Muehlbauer MJ, van der Westhuizen J, Mathew JP, Schwinn DA, Glower DD, Newgard CB, Podgoreanu MV.(2009). Metabolomic profiling reveals distinct patterns of myocardial substrate use in humans with coronary artery disease or left ventricular dysfunction during surgical ischemia/reperfusion. *Circulation* 119:1736-1746.

[32] Zheng X, Shen J, Liu Q, Wang S, Cheng Y, Qu H. (2009). Plasma fatty acids metabolic profiling analysis of coronary heart disease based on GC-MS and pattern recognition. *J. Pharm. Biomed. Anal.* 49:481-486.

[33] Mayr M, Yusuf S, Weir G, Chung YL, Mayr U, Yin X, Ladroue C, Madhu B, Roberts N, De Souza A, Fredericks S, Stubbs M, Griffiths JR, Jahangiri M, Xu Q, Camm AJ.(2008). Combined metabolomic and proteomic analysis of human atrial fibrillation. *J. Am. Coll. Cardiol.* 51:585-594.

[34] Barba I, de Leon G, Martin E, Cuevas A, Aguade S, Candell-Riera J, Barrabés JA, Garcia-Dorado D.(2008). Nuclear magnetic resonance-based metabolomics predicts exercise-induced ischemia in patients with suspected coronary artery disease. *Magn. Reson. Med.* 60:27-32.

[35] Kirschenlohr HL, Griffin JL, Clarke SC, Rhydwen R, Grace AA, Schofield PM, Brindle KM, Metcalfe JC. (2006). Proton NMR analysis of plasma is a weak predictor of coronary artery disease. *Nat. Med.* 2:705-710.

[36] Sabatine MS, Liu E, Morrow DA, Heller E, McCarroll R, Wiegand R, Berriz GF, Roth FP, Gerszten RE.(2005). Metabolomic identification of novel biomarkers of myocardial ischemia. *Circulation* 112:3868-3875.

Index

G

H

I

N

O

P

Q

R

S

T

U

V

W